The Ultimate Dash Diet Guide

2021 EDITION

TABLE OF CONTENTS

CHAPTER 14 DESSERT RECIPES

CHAPTER 15 28 DAY MEAL PLAN

CONCLUSION

Introduction

With the vast amount of diet programs out there, it could be hard to identify one designed to fit the body type and lifestyle of yours. Thankfully, there are some that appear to work on a broad level for people even in case their objectives are somewhat different. The DASH Diet, for example, is a health regiment which was initially created for individuals with hypertension or maybe high blood pressure. Doctors and nutritionists realized that blood pressure level increased in the patients whenever they consumed sodium and thus DASH was developed to place their people over a low sodium diet plan.

The advantage of the DASH Diet, nonetheless, is that the individuals noticed they dropped a few pounds along with decreasing the blood pressure. Since that time, it's been the most popular diet program to come through since the 1990s. Among the other factors to pick the DASH Diet could be the adaptability that it provides to those who make it part of their daily routine. For starters, there's a choice when it involves the salt levels: for those who would like a simple decrease in the sodium intake, they can choose the regular amount of intake of 2,300 milligrams. For those who wish to clear away a substantial amount of sodium from the daily intake of theirs, their use is lowered to 1,500 mg each day. Once again, that offers some flexibility.

The DASH Diet is additionally not entirely restrictive, as a few diets are identified to be. An excellent benefit for this diet is the reality that it can be achieved in 2 phases. The very 1st stage will last around 2 weeks and also during this particular time the dieter must stay away from starchy food and sugars almost as possible. This's done so that the maximum amount of abdominal fat is lost over the first two weeks. In the 2nd stage, several healthy starches are re-introduced to the diet plan together with the idea that the body will by now have the boosted metabolic rate to manage them. Dieters still lose some weight and are urged to stick to Phase 2 almost as you can for the long haul.

Another benefit for this diet is the fact that Phase 2 is very suitable for the eating patterns that individuals now have by relying on basic switches, like empty to whole cereals and snack foods which are loaded with protein. There's not a great deal of sacrifice, though a big benefit when all has been said and done.

Is the DASH Diet Right for You?

If you are afflicted by hypertension or even have a high risk of developing blood pressure troubles, the DASH weight loss program is very healthy for you. Actually, with its diet techniques, the DASH Diet is a superb plan for everybody.

As a result of the growing problem of morbid obesity in the US and anywhere else, metabolic syndrome is on the rise. In case you're drastically overweight or have a big waistline and extra abdominal fat, you might have metabolic syndrome or perhaps in danger of creating it.

The best part is that metabolic syndrome is fully or partially reversed with combining physical exercise and a DASH style diet. Experts have found that results that are similar are possible for those with type two diabetes.

But what in case you're not impacted by these illnesses? What in case you're simply searching for a healthful way to lose some weight and possibly stop these conditions down the road?

In case you're thinking about the DASH Diet for preventative reasons and weight loss, then you're more likely to think it is being an appealing choice for long-term health. The DASH Diet suggests you consume a wide variety of food from all of the food organizations, manuals you through the method of determining the ideal calorie intake and oftentimes improves participants' metabolism and energy. While many other diet programs propose unhealthy eating patterns as well as starvation, DASH's nutritious food-centric method is a realistic and excellent option for several.

Added advantages of the DASH Diet:

• You are more likely to find DASH friendly meal choices when eating at restaurants or maybe a friend's home.

• The realistic ways of DASH ensure it is easier to keep the weight once you have achieved the ideal weight of yours.

• You have the choice to pick a sodium level which is suitable for you.

• The DASH eating habit outlines just how you are able to maximize or even decrease the caloric intake as the activity level of yours as well as body mass change.

• It is easy to adjust popular dishes to fit the DASH Diet plan.

It is not difficult to see exactly why millions of individuals have considered selecting the DASH Diet plan to improve their health and lose excess fat and weight. With this guide, you will have all that you have to achieve success on the diet.

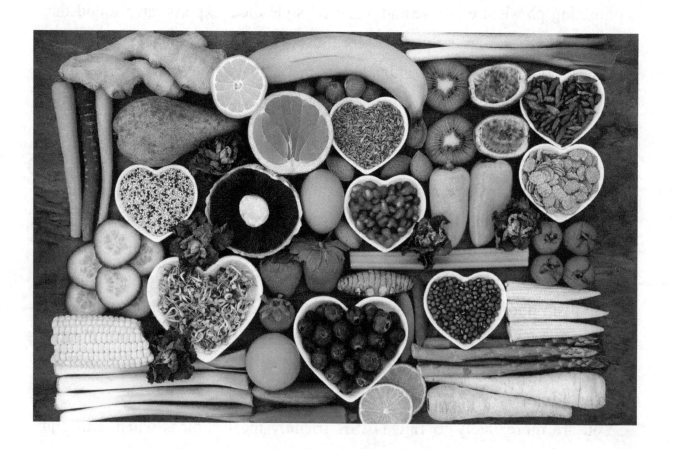

Chapter 1   About Dash Diet

This is the 9th record time DASH diet was among the best diets in the world according to the health report "US News".

From 2010, the DASH diet was selected annually as the number 1 among the most popular nutrition systems; in 2018 it won first place along with the Mediterranean diet, while for 2019 it is recommended immediately after it.

The "US News Health Report" ranking in the "Best Diet" category is created with the participation of over 20 experts, including dietitians, dietary consultants and doctors specializing in, among others in slimming and treating heart disease or diabetes.

As part of it, 41 diets were assessed for features such as protection against civilization diseases, ease of use, the effect on weight loss and the ability to maintain a lower weight. In terms of impact on health, the DASH diet scored 4.8 points out of 5!

The DASH diet is suitable for people of all ages, providing numerous beneficial effects and a drop in blood pressure after just 2 weeks!

Diet Dash - Dietary Approaches to Stop Hypertension

The name of the DASH diet comes from the name of the study in which it was evaluated - it was titled "Dietary Approach to Stop Hypertension" - "Dietary Approaches to Stop Hypertension". They were carried out more than 20 years ago in support of the American National Institute of Heart, Lung and Blood-forming System (NHLBI), which is the body of the National Institute of Health (NIH).

Because untreated hypertension increases the risk of developing heart disease, heart attack and stroke, the right nutritional strategy was to help reduce the risk of developing it. The diet has proved extremely effective and to this day there are more discoveries about its beneficial effects on health.

It has been proven, among others, that the DASH diet helps prevent the development of hypertension facilitates the improvement of an abnormal blood lipidogram, reduces the risk of developing cardiovascular diseases and type 2 diabetes, as well as general mortality, contributing to prolonged life.

The high effectiveness of the DASH diet is related to its design, reminiscent of the Mediterranean style diet on which it was modeled. However, the beneficial effect is mainly due to the fact that sodium intake is reduced and potassium, magnesium and calcium doses are increased.

It is possible thanks to limiting the consumption of industrial food, especially of animal origin, and increasing the number of greens and other unprocessed plant products, especially cereals.

Dash Diet Definition

DASH (Dietary Approaches to Stop Hypertension) has been designed by American researchers to reduce or prevent hypertension.

It is rich in fruits, vegetables and whole grains, as well as low-fat or fat-free dairy products, fish, poultry, beans, seeds and nuts. Fats and sugars are very limited.

DASH is a flexible meal plan that focuses on natural foods such as vegetables, fruits, whole grains, non-fat or low-fat dairy products, fish, chicken, beans, nuts, and vegetable oils (such as olive oil). All ingredients are effective in promoting health, including diet.

The DASH diet was not originally made to lose weight. But it is clear that factors that affect blood pressure (processed foods, trans fatty acids, excess sugar, etc.) also affect body weight. Studies have shown that people who continued DASH diets lost more weight in 8-24 weeks than other low-calorie diets.

The abbreviation of DASH is the acronym of Dietary Approaches to Stop Hypertension which means that it is a dietary program based on dietary results recommended by the expert group of a famous institution in 1997 to lower blood pressure.

The DASH healthy diet is a certified treatment for hypertension, heart disease and kidney disease even without any medical help. Hypertension is also called the silent killer that has no previous symptom or warning.

The DASH diet completely emphasizes the correct nutrition of foods with the portion size and the right amount of nutritional value.

This diet plan is a combined plant-based diet that should be rich in whole grains, fruits, vegetables, nuts, seeds, meat, nuts etc. It is also rich in dietary fiber, potassium, calcium, protein and magnesium.

But it must be low in sodium, cholesterol, fatty dairy products. This perfect combination of diet is highly recommendable for the person who wants to prevent or control hypertension which also reduces the risk of contracting heart disease.

The functionality of these properly planned diets is classified into a logical category based on seven types of security: easy to follow, high nutritional value, short term weight loss results, effective and preventive management of diabetes and various heart conditions.

More on Dash Diet

The DASH project compared 3 different types of diet:

1 group followed normal eating habits; the second group saw the increase in the quantities of fruit and vegetables, while the third group had to follow the DASH dietary plan.

The results showed that both the second and the third group were able to reduce blood pressure, but in the case of the DASH diet this result was achieved in just 2 weeks.

The second study, called DASH-Sodium, instead set itself the goal of verifying how lower sodium levels in the diet could affect blood pressure.

The study participants were divided into 2 macro-categories (one followed the DASH plan of the first project, the other the normal supply) and each macro-category was then divided into 3 further categories based on the sodium levels in the feed: over 3300 mg, about 2400 mg and 1500 mg of sodium.

The research results showed that a reduction in sodium levels showed a reduction in blood pressure for both macro-categories, and the greatest reduction occurred in the 1500mg-plane DASH combination.

DASH diet has been classified as the best and healthiest against hypertension and diabetes for 3 consecutive years.

It has been shown to reduce blood pressure and cholesterol, as it is also excellent to follow in the presence of some diseases, but it is ideal for keeping hypertension under control.

If your blood pressure rises above 120/80 even slightly, you may already notice some side effects.

The more blood pressure deviates from optimal values, the greater the risk to our health. Researchers began to investigate the causes of high blood pressure by analyzing single elements, such as calcium and magnesium, but none of those studies was able to arrive at certain results.

In America, there were then two key research supported by the NHLBI.

The first study, called DASH, analyzed the influence of each food on blood pressure and discovered that blood pressure was reduced following a diet low in saturated fats and cholesterol, and emphasizing instead the intake of low fruit, vegetables and products of fat.

They then elaborated on a dietary plan, DASH precisely, which also included the intake of products based on durum wheat, poultry fish and hazelnuts, while limiting red meat, sweets and sugary drinks.

The plan was also rich in magnesium, potassium and calcium, as well as protein and fiber.

Dash Diet Start Up

The DASH diet was originally developed over twenty years ago at Harvard University in the United States and its main purpose was to control hypertension, a widespread disease in the adult population and with serious consequences.

The DASH diet, thanks to the foods of which it is rich, presents a high quantity of vitamins, calcium, magnesium, potassium, fibers and polyphenols.

It is a diet rich in fruits, vegetables, mostly whole grains and low-fat dairy products. Dried fruits, legumes, seeds, fish and white meat are also present in moderate quantities, while foods such as red meat, fried foods and desserts are limited.

The first of the research concerning the DASH diet was carried out on 459 adults, with systolic pressure below 160 mmHg and diastolic blood pressure between 80 and 95 mmHg.

About 27% of the participants suffered from hypertension; about 50% were female and 60% were of African-American origin.

In the research three different diets were compared:

- The first included foods similar to those normally taken by the American population;

- The second was identical to the first, with the addition of fruit and vegetables;

- The third was the DASH diet.

All three diets included a daily sodium intake of 3,000 mg; none were vegetarians nor did they provide common foods in specific ethnic traditions.

The results were sensational. Those who followed both the diet with fruit and vegetable supplementation and the dash diet managed to lower the pressure, but it was the dash diet that achieved the best results, especially among people with hypertension.

In addition, the pressure decreased almost immediately, within two weeks of starting the diet.

The second research concerning the dash diet focused on the effects of reduced sodium consumption on blood pressure: the participants, divided into two groups, followed the dash diet and another diet that reflected normal Western diet, respectively.

In this second research 412 people were involved, to whom one of the two groups was randomly assigned, and who then had to stick to one of the three sodium levels expected for a month:

- The high level, that is the one consumed by the majority of Americans and equal to 3,300 mg per day,

- The average one, equal to 2,300 mg a day

- And the low one, equal to 1,500 mg a day.

The results showed that, by decreasing sodium consumption, the pressure subsided, regardless of the diet followed.

Furthermore, at each level, the pressure was lower in those who had followed the dash diet. The most significant decreases in blood pressure occurred among patients who followed the dash diet with a sodium intake of 1,500 milligrams per day.

Those who already suffered from hypertension previously experienced the sharpest decreases, but even those with prehypertension experienced significant decreases in blood pressure.

Jointly considered these two kinds of research shows that it is important to decrease the consumption of sodium, regardless of the diet that is followed.

The winning combination, however, is represented by the dash diet and the decrease in salt and sodium consumption.

Effect of Dash Diet

According to research conducted in 2017, the results of which are described in the Journal of American College of Cardiology, a low-sodium diet rich in heart-beneficial products, such as DASH, can lower too high blood pressure as well as commonly used drugs.

According to the Hypertension magazine, patients with elevated blood pressure following the DASH diet for 8 weeks resulted in a reduction in systolic pressure by an average of 6 mm Hg, and diastolic pressure by 3 mm Hg.

In hypertensive patients, the decreases in systolic and diastolic blood pressure were 11 and 6 mm Hg, respectively. The body weight of the subjects did not change.

The fact that the use of the DASH diet allows similar or even greater drops in blood pressure than when taking popular medications has been confirmed by the research discussed in the Journal of the American College of Cardiology.

They tested 2 versions of the diet - standard (2,300 mg sodium per day) and low-sodium (1,500 mg sodium per day). After 4 weeks, the reduction in blood pressure was higher compared to the high- sodium control diet, the higher the initial value of systolic pressure in patients:

above 150 mm Hg - 21 mm Hg less with low-sodium DASH, and 11 mm Hg less - with standard; 140-149 mm Hg - 10 mm Hg less with low-sodium and standard DASH;

130-139 mm Hg -7 mm Hg less with low sodium DASH and 4 mm Hg less with standard, up to 130 mm Hg - 5 mm Hg less with low sodium DASH, 4 mm Hg less with standard.

The DASH diet version richer in fat thanks to the use of full-fat dairy products proved to be as effective in reducing high blood pressure as the standard one - results from CHORI studies.

The results of which have been described in the American Journal of Clinical Nutrition, with the modified menu being slightly poorer in simple carbohydrates, incl. from fruit juices. After 3 weeks, it reduced the level of triglycerides and large and medium VLDL cholesterol molecules more effectively than the standard version of the diet.

The introduction of the DASH diet protects women against the development of heart disease, which was confirmed in studies from the "Archives of Internal Medicine".

Participants using menus that most met the diet requirements by 24% were less likely to get coronary heart disease and by 18% they had a fewer stroke. Lower levels of C-reactive protein and interleukin-6 have been found in their blood, which are indicators of inflammation in the body.

The DASH diet reduces the risk of gout - a painful inflammatory disease of the joints (usually the big toe) caused by the accumulation of uric acid crystals in them (another place where they can accumulate are the kidneys - the effect is kidney stones).

Statistics show that almost 75 percent. Patients with gout also have hypertension, and in more than 60 percent. Metabolic syndrome is found.

In a survey lasting over 26 years conducted on over 44,000 men aged 40 and over, the rarer the occurrence of the disease was confirmed, the closer the daily diet was to the DASH recommendations.

Adhering to the recommendations of the DASH diet also reduces the incidence of depression in the elderly, which results from studies presented in 2018 at the annual congress of the American Academy of Neurology.

During the 6.5-year period under study, it was shown that a diet closer to the ideal DASH recommendations reduces the risk of depression by up to 11 percent, and the more it resembles a Western-style menu, the more it promotes the development of this disease.

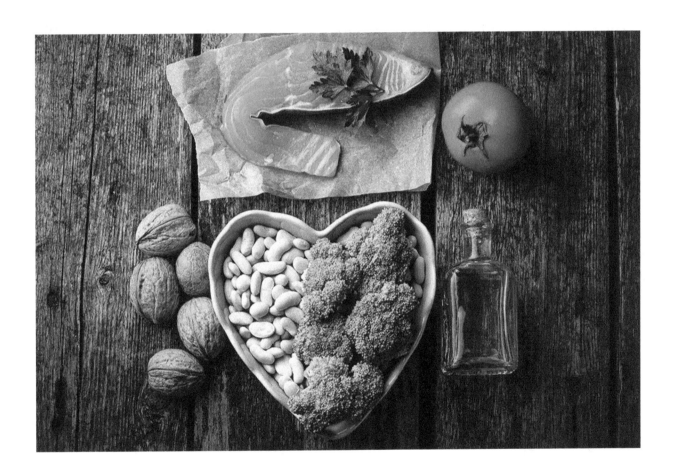

Habit Checklist of Dash Diet

DASH diet is a new diet and a diet that you should follow throughout your life. If you don't follow it for several days, don't be discouraged and go back to the "right path" and continue to pursue your food goals.

Ask yourself why you are tempted. Was there a party? Did you feel stress due to work or family life? Find the cause of the temporary departure from the route and resume immediately after the dash diet.

Don't worry too much. Sooner or later, all those who follow the diet will seduce themselves, especially when they are still in the running-in phase. Remember that lifestyle changes are a process that can last a long time.

Ask yourself if you have done too much at once. In many cases, people trying to change their lifestyles are overkill. Try to change a few things at once. The change will be slower, but it is certainly the best way to do it.

Divide the process into many small steps. Doing so will not only invite you to do too much at once, but also make it easier to change. A single difficult task can be broken up into smaller and simpler steps and created very easily.

Keep a diary. Use the agenda to keep track of what you eat and what you do. This makes it easier to understand where the problem is. Keep a diary for several days.

You may find yourself used to eat fatty foods while watching TV. In this case, you can start by keeping an alternative snack low in fat.

A diary can also help you determine if you have a balanced diet and have enough physical activity.

Dos and Cons of the Dash Diet

Among the DOS we find:

• Lowering cholesterol and high blood pressure

• lose weight

• The organism is purified

• Prevent tumor

• Against the onset of diabetes

• Helps combat moisture retention

• It's a simple meal that doesn't require much time

• Vegetarians can also practice

• Also suitable for people suffering from celiac disease and lactose intolerance

In the CONS we find:

• Give up sweets that are healthy but not easy for everyone

There are no special contraindications for the Dash diet. Obviously it is highly recommended not to eat without medical supervision

Chapter 2   What is the Dash Diet

Most as of late, researchers took a gander at the DASH diets impact on cholesterol esteems too. It turns out, those hoping to control blood weight and lower cholesterol levels have considerably more motivation to attempt the DASH; the DASH diet essentially lowered aggregate and LDL-cholesterol (alluded to as the "awful" cholesterol) levels in subjects with marginal high and high cholesterol.

DASH Diet - Real-Life Solutions

Avocado plunge, for instance, is a standout amongst the most famous Dash diets there is today, because of its helpful and reasonable arrangement. Avocado, an exceptionally rich source of monosaturated fat and lutein, (cancer prevention agents that assistance protects vision), is among the numerous natural products that are highly-suggested for Dash diet. In this recipe, avocado must be squashed and hollowed, blended with fat-free acrid cream, onion, and hot sauce. This plunge shall be eaten with tortilla chips or cut vegetables. From this dish, a person can get a total of 65 calories, 2 grams protein, 5 grams total fat, 4 grams sugar, 172 milligrams potassium and 31 milligrams calcium. From this, we can infer that a person is sustained a considerable amount of necessary supplements, fundamental for maintaining a well-adjusted diet that is useful for the heart.

In just 14 days, a Dash diet follower will encounter ordinary circulatory strain, with fewer inclinations to eat in-between meals, the real guilty party of weight gain. The Dash diet program additionally teaches individuals to determine the right amount of food intake, the necessary exercise to perform according to age and movement level. Dash instructs and motivates - one of the important reasons why people find it simple to stick to the diet.

Additionally, the diet does not require us to quit any pretense of anything significant in our usual diet, instead, it causes us to make a procedure of adjusting to little changes so we can effectively support ourselves.

The Best Diabetes Diet

After some time, many diabetes diet - that is, diets created with the end goal of helping people with diabetes better deal with their diabetes, have been created, had their prime and unobtrusively passed away into bright retirement. Many however remain solid and just as popular as when they were first presented. However, how effective however are these diets.

With the list seeming to develop longer constantly, it frequently leaves a bewildered open pondering where to start. So I chose to do review of the most popular diets currently on the market and toward the finish of that review two diets came through as exceptional entertainers for helping people deal with their diabetes. One of them being the DASH diet. What follows is a brief of what I found out about that diet. However, before we go into that, one might need to ask, what precisely makes up a decent Diabetic diet? The following in this way are just a portion of those components.

1. It will be low on carbohydrates or if nothing else accommodate a method for either offsetting the sugar through the course of the day or "consuming" off the overabundance, as, through exercise.

2. It ought to be high in dietary fiber which has been demonstrated to have numerous health benefits like having a low glycemic record and lowering the probabilities for sicknesses like coronary illness and so on.

3. Low in salt. Salt can prompt hypertension-that is high blood pressure, so chopping it down is a must

4. Low in fat. Since fat or foods effectively converted to fat like sugars can prompt the individual getting to be overweight-a risk factor for diabetes, usually essential for such sustenance to have a low-fat substance.

5. A decent diabetic diet ought to endeavor to meet the recommended daily allowance for potassium. Potassium is important because it can turn around the negative effects on the circulatory framework that salt has.

Anyway that isn't the extent that its advantages go. The diet has additionally been observed to be similarly efficacious as a diabetes diet. In fact, in a review of 35 diets did by US News and World report recently it turned out joint first with The Biggest Loser diet as the best diabetes diet. Mirroring much of the advice offered by the American Diabetes Association, it has been shown to show both diabetes avoidance and control characteristics.

On counteractive action, it has been shown to enable individuals to get in shape and furthermore keep it off. Since being overweight is a major risk factor for creating Type 2 diabetes, this quality shows it off as an extraordinary diabetes diet alternative.

What's more, the risk factors related with metabolic disorder, a condition which builds the odds of creating diabetes is likewise diminished by a blend of the DASH diet and calorie restriction. As regards control, the results of a small study published in a 2011 edition of Diabetes Care uncovered that Type 2 diabetics following two months on DASH had decreased their dimensions of A1C and their fasting blood sugar.

Also the diet has been observed to be more adaptable than most, a fact that would make it simpler to follow and adjustable, to empower it agree to a specialist's dietary advice to his diabetic patient.

Another favorable position offered by this diet is the dimension of its adjustment to dietary rules. Light as it might appear, this is actually important because a few diets place a restriction on specific foods, along these lines leaving the individual possibly insufficient in specific nutrients and minerals.

A breakdown of this congruity demonstrates that where fat is concerned, the diet satisfactorily falls inside the 20 to 35 percent of daily calories recommended by the administration. It likewise meets the 10 percent maximum limit dispensed to immersed fat by falling admirably below that. It likewise meets the recommended amount of proteins and carbohydrates.

Where salt is concerned, it has rule feast tops for this mineral. Both for the recommended daily maximum of 2,300 mg and in case you're African-American, are 51 years or more seasoned or have hypertension, diabetes or unending kidney illness, the 1,500 mg limit.

Different nutrients are enough dealt with additionally by this diet. Thus the recommended daily intake of 22 to 34 grams' fiber for adults is very much accommodated by this diet. So too is potassium, a nutrient that is set apart for its ability to counter salts blood pressure raising characteristics, diminish the risk of creating kidney stones and furthermore decline bone misfortune. Impressively so because of the difficulty in normally procuring the recommended daily intake-4,700 mg or the equivalent of eating 11 bananas every day.

Recommended daily intake of Vitamin D for adults who don't get enough sunlight is penciled down at 15 mg. However, the diet falls just short of this, it is recommended that this can be effectively made up by state a nutrient D invigorated grain.

Calcium so vital for solid bones and teeth, blood vessel generation and muscle work is additionally enough dealt with by the diet. The administration's recommendation of between 1,000 mg to 1300 mg is met here effectively with no affectation or graces. The equivalent goes for

Vitamin B-12. The administration's recommendation is 2.4 mg. The diets arrangement is 6.7.

What You Need To Know

There is a specific eating plan that has been proven to bring down hypertension or high pulse. This diet is known as the DASH or Dietary Approaches to Stop Hypertension.

What is DASH diet?

The DASH diet is a consequence of clinical examinations directed by researchers of the National Heart, Lung and Blood Institute (NHLBI). The researchers discovered that a diet high in potassium, magnesium, calcium, protein and fiber, and low in fat and cholesterol can radically decrease high circulatory strain.

The investigation demonstrated that a diet rich in vegetables, fruits and low-fat dairy items had a major impact in diminishing hypertension. It additionally demonstrated that the DASH diet produces fast outcomes, sometimes in as meager as about fourteen days in the wake of beginning the diet.

The DASH diet additionally underlines on three significant supplements: magnesium, calcium and potassium. These minerals are thought to help lessen high circulatory strain. A normal 2,000-calorie diet contains 500 milligrams of magnesium, 4.7 grams of potassium and 1.2 grams of calcium.

Doing the DASH Diet

Following the DASH diet is exceptionally simple and takes little time in the choice and planning of dinners. Foods rich in fats and cholesterol are maintained a strategic distance from.

Since the foods you eat in a DASH diet are high in fiber content, it is suggested that you gradually increment your utilization of fiber-rich sustenance to evade loose bowels and other stomach related issues. You can bit by bit increment your fiber intake by eating an additional serving of fruits and vegetables in each dinner.

If you choose to eat meat, limit your utilization to just six ounces per day, which is comparable in size to a deck of cards. You can likewise eat more vegetables, cereals, pasta and beans into your meat dishes. Low-fat milk or skim milk is likewise a great source of protein without the excess fat and cholesterol.

For snacks, you can attempt canned or dried fruits, just as crisp ones. There are additionally healthy snack alternatives for those on the DASH diet, for example, graham saltines, unsalted nuts and low-fat yogurt.

It's Easy to DASH

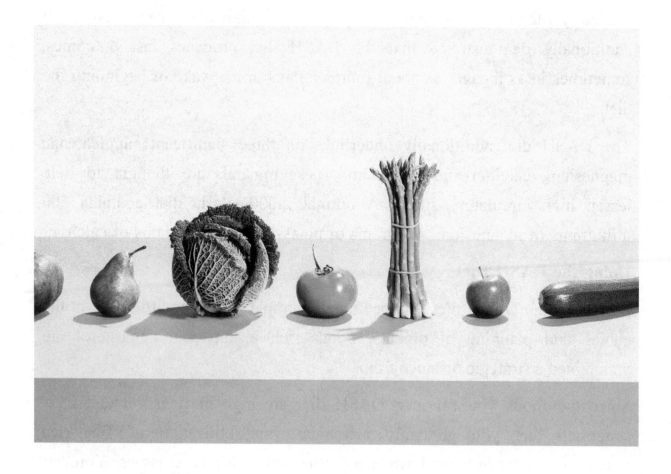

Chapter 3   Principles of Dash Diet

Whole Grains and Starchy Vegetables

Whole grains and starchy vegetables are good sources of fiber, helping to slow the absorption of glucose in the blood. Packed with vitamins and minerals, these foods should always be chosen over refined and processed carbohydrates. Whole grains include brown rice, barley, farro, quinoa, oats, and whole-grain pasta; starchy vegetables include potatoes and sweet potatoes.

Servings: Aim for four to six servings daily. One serving equates to one-half cup of cooked grains, one slice of whole grain bread, or one medium-size sweet potato.

Helpful Tips and Tricks: Short on time or don't want to cook? No problem! Instead of making a pot of brown rice, you can look for precooked, frozen whole grains in your grocer's freezer aisle.

Fruits and Vegetables

Fruits and vegetables are a vital part of the Mediterranean DASH diet. Full of vitamins, minerals, and antioxidants, these are nutrient powerhouses in our day-to-day life. These fiber-rich foods help us feel full and satisfied, support lower blood pressure and weight management, and help ward off a variety of diseases. Be sure to eat plenty of alliums, such as garlic, onions, and leeks, as well as a good amount of crucifers, including broccoli, cauliflower, and Brussels sprouts, on a weekly basis.

Servings: Aim to consume at least four to five servings of vegetables and three servings of fruit daily. One serving equates to one-half cup of fruit or cooked vegetables, or one cup of raw leafy greens.

Helpful Tips and Tricks: Fresh and frozen will be your go-to foundation, but canned and packed in water or natural juices are great to keep on hand as a backup option. And don't forget dried fruit, a great addition to your yogurt or oatmeal or sprinkled on top of a salad!

Building a Plate

Traditional Mediterranean cuisine is enjoyed as part of a balanced lifestyle, which includes a sustainable approach to eating well. The cornerstone of any healthy diet is a properly proportioned plate. Fruits and vegetables are eaten in plenty, while meats, sweet treats, and wine are enjoyed in moderation. A balanced plate should be one-half non-starchy vegetables, one-quarter whole grains or starchy vegetables, and one-quarter lean protein.

Lean Proteins: Animal and Plant

Lean proteins encompass both animal and plant-based protein sources. In the Mediterranean DASH diet, we place a heavier emphasis on fish and shellfish, with smaller portions of eggs, lean poultry, and meat. When selecting beef, pork, and other animal protein, look for leaner cuts, such as loin and round. These cuts of meat are flavorful and easy to prepare while also being lower in saturated fat. Eggs and poultry are largely excellent choices as well.

Plant-based protein sources are superstars. They are high in fiber and complex carbohydrates while being low in fat. They are also sources of other key minerals and nutrients, such as potassium, magnesium, folate, and iron. Plant-based proteins include beans and legumes, such as lentils, peas, and soy. For our purposes, nuts and seeds will also be part of this category, contributing lean protein and healthy fats.

Servings: Aim to get up to six ounces per day of lean meat, poultry, or seafood. Think of a three-ounce portion as the size of a deck of playing cards. Try to get two to three servings of seafood on a weekly basis. Aim for four to five servings of nuts, seeds, beans, and legumes per week. One serving is about one-half cup cooked beans or legumes, three ounces of tempeh or tofu, and one-third cup of nuts and seeds.

Helpful Tips and Tricks: Keep low-sodium versions of canned tuna, salmon, and beans on hand to help get meals on the table quickly and easily.

Healthy Fats and Oils

Olives and olive oil are staples in the Mediterranean DASH diet, known for their heart-healthy monounsaturated fat content and anti-inflammatory properties. For a more neutral-flavored oil, canola oil is a good choice.

Another great source of healthy fat is the avocado. Research has shown that the high levels of oleic acid found in avocados help decrease LDL, the "bad" cholesterol, and boost HDL, the "good" cholesterol.

Servings: Aim for two to three servings of fats and oils daily. One serving equates to one teaspoon of oil or one-quarter of an avocado.

Helpful Tips and Tricks: Making your own salad dressing is a great way to incorporate flavorful, low-sodium versions into your daily routine. Use empty jam or nut butter jars to make larger batches, which will keep in the refrigerator for a couple of weeks.

Low-Fat Dairy

Low-fat dairy foods such as cheese and yogurt are foundational foods in the Mediterranean DASH diet. The dairy group contributes important nutrients, including calcium, vitamin D, and potassium. Studies have shown that fermented dairy products, such as yogurt and some cheeses, have an inverse relationship with cardiovascular disease and type 2 diabetes. There is some evidence that eating fermented dairy foods may help fight inflammation associated with the development of heart disease.

Servings: Aim to consume two to three servings of low-fat dairy daily. One serving equates to one cup of nonfat or low-fat plain yogurt (includes Greek yogurt) or one-and-a-half ounces of cheese.

Helpful Tips and Tricks: Have a hankering for tuna salad? Use plain yogurt in place of mayonnaise to add protein, flavor, and richness without the added saturated fat and calories. Yogurt can also be added to foods like soup and oatmeal to increase the protein content and add creaminess without using butter or heavy cream.

Limited Added Sugar

The Mediterranean DASH diet naturally decreases sugar intake without making you feel deprived in any way. Dessert and sweet treats can still be part of your weekly routine, but with a focus on natural sources of sugar, such as fruit sugars, honey, and maple syrup.

Servings: Aim to limit sugar to five or fewer servings per week. One serving size equals one tablespoon of maple syrup or honey, or one-half cup of ice cream or frozen yogurt.

Helpful Tips and Tricks: Try adding fresh or dried fruit and a teaspoon of jam to a bowl of oatmeal or yogurt in place of sugar.

Limited Sodium

Many foods naturally contain some sodium. However, much of the sodium many of us consume is added to foods, making it too easy for most people to over consume. You can find it hiding in most processed foods and often added in huge quantities to restaurant meals. Excessive sodium intake is one of the main drivers of high blood pressure. Using less salt, and instead relying on herbs and spices to add bold flavor to foods, is a key component of the Mediterranean DASH diet.

Servings: Aim to consume between 1,500 and 2,300 milligrams of sodium per day. For reference, one-quarter teaspoon of kosher salt equals about 500 milligrams of sodium.

Helpful Tips and Tricks: Reach for herbs and spices to create depth of flavor, adding salt in small amounts. You can always add salt, but once it's there you cannot take it away!

The recipes included in the Mediterranean DASH diet follow these guidelines:

Snacks, sides, and desserts: ≤300 milligrams of sodium

Entrées and meals: ≤570 milligrams of sodium

Sneaky Sodium

To keep your sodium intake in check, it is essential to be able to properly read a food label. The first step is to become familiar with portion sizing (i.e., if you eat two servings worth of a food, you double your sodium intake). As with sugar, it is important to recognize the difference between naturally occurring sodium in foods and added salt. Some foods, like celery, beets, and milk, organically contain sodium in low levels, which supply our bodies with electrolytes. Added salt is salt added during cooking and processing, and this is what accounts for most of our daily sodium intake. Examples of foods typically loaded with added salt include canned foods, cured and deli-style meats, cheeses, frozen prepared meals, soups, chips, and condiments. To help prevent excessive sodium intake, look for foods labeled "no salt added," "low-sodium," or "sodium-free." When using canned items, such as beans and lentils, rinse well with water prior to using. And try using garlic, citrus juice, herbs, and spices for flavor before reaching for the saltshaker.

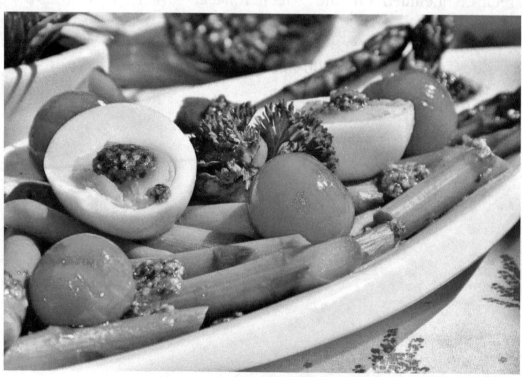

Chapter 4   DASH Diet Leads to a Healthier Kidney

The DASH Diet is supported by the National Kidney Foundation. Hypertension is related to kidney diseases. Since the DASH Diet helps decrease the blood pressure level, it can also help reduce the onset of kidney diseases. The reduced intake of salt and other Sodium-rich foods can help reduce the formation of kidney stones.

DASH   Diet   and Cholesterol/Heart/Disease/Osteoporosis/Stroke

The DASH Diet comes with a lot of benefits for the body. It is also known to lower down cholesterol level, improve heart health, prevent stroke, and osteoporosis. Because it promotes the consumption of good fats and fatty acid, it can help increase the number of low-density lipoproteins (LDL) in the blood. Good fats also help prevent inflammation. It protects major organs, particularly the cardiovascular system, thereby improving heart health. Having better heart health also prevents the likelihood of stroke. And since the DASH Diet promotes the consumption of micronutrients, including Calcium, it can also help improve bone strength and avoid the early onset of osteoporosis.

Hypertension: How Does Diet Come into Play and Why DASH Diet Works?

Food plays a vital role in the development of hypertension. Studies showed that consumption of foods rich in Sodium (salt), particularly processed food, can increase the likelihood of developing hypertension. But can diet alone help stabilize blood pressure levels? Researchers from the NIH noted that dietary interventions play vital roles in improving the condition of people suffering from different situations. Dietary change can decrease the systolic blood pressure level by about 6 to 11 mmHg. This means that by following the right diet regimen and omitting foods that are not helpful to the blood pressure level can bring relief to hypertensive people.

The DASH Diet was developed by expert nutritionists and has undergone several trials to prove that it can really benefit by reducing the systolic pressure. In fact, the reduction of the systolic blood pressure was observed not only among hypertensive individuals but also those who have normal blood pressure levels.

Preparing to Embrace the DASH Diet

Tips for Planning Your DASH Diet

The DASH Diet is one of the easiest ways to maintain your healthy lifestyle, thus it does not take rocket science for you to be able to follow and achieve your health goals with this diet. When planning to do the DASH Diet, there are some things that you need to consider first. Below are important tips for planning your DASH Diet.

• Make small changes: Remember that this particular diet regimen encourages you to make diet changes by eating whole foods. Making small changes allow you to adjust to this regimen easily. You can do this by gradually making changes in your diet. For instance, you can add more serving of vegetables every meal or substitute unhealthy dressings with healthier condiments.

• Limit your intake of meat: Start limiting the amount of meat that you are going to take in. If you are currently eating large amounts of meat, you can start cutting back at least two servings every day.

• Start avoiding full-fat options: Start avoiding full-fat options once you start planning to do the DASH Diet. It is easier to omit foods that are not allowed for this particular diet, especially when you started restricting yourself earlier in the first place.

• Practice smart shopping: Shopping is one of the biggest aspects of the DASH Diet. Since your shopping will be restricted to buying whole fresh food, you need to learn how to read food labels and choose items that do not contain any unnecessary additives, particularly salt. This is also the time when you start removing processed foods from your shopping list.

• Start cooking healthy: When you cook your food, try learning how to cook without too much or no salt at all. This may be challenging for you, but you can try experimenting with different salt-free flavorings, herbs, and spices.

•	Eat out less often: If you love to eat out all the time, try to minimize your dinner trips once you have started with the DASH Diet. This is especially true if you are still getting the hang of this diet. The problem with eating out is that most restaurants either use too much salt when flavoring their food. If you cannot help but eat out, ask the restaurant to prepare food without added salt or MSG.

•	Plan your meals ahead: Another tip to make you successful in your DASH Diet is to plan your meals ahead. Planning your meals weekly is a great way to stick to this diet. A weekly meal plan will also serve as your guide on when to eat and what to eat. This will help you avoid over snacking or eating foods that you are not supposed to eat.

The DASH Diet Food Pyramid

The DASH Diet is a very straight-forward diet regimen, but it still helps especially for starters like you to have a guide. This is where the DASH Diet food pyramid comes in. The DASH Diet pyramid is just like your usual food guide, but it indicates what types of food you can eat for this particular diet regimen with specific serving amounts for a 2000-calorie daily diet. The food pyramid is also carefully designed to reduce the total fat in food choices.

The food items that are listed at the bottom of the pyramid are the fruits and vegetables. They should be consumed at 8 to 10 servings daily. This is followed by whole grains. Both the low-fat and meats are at the third tier of the pyramid that means you need to consume less of it. The fourth level of the pyramid includes beans, nuts, and seeds. While sweets belong to the top of the pyramid and should be taken with fewer servings weekly. If you notice, there are only three types of food groups that are included in the food pyramid. Below is a short summary of the types of food that you are allowed to eat under the DASH Diet.

• Carbohydrates: Carbohydrates is sourced from different types of foods, including fruits, vegetables, grains, nuts, and seeds. They contain starch and cellulose. The DASH Diet encourages the consumption of healthy starches not only to supply energy for the body but to provide the body with protective micronutrients. Healthy sources of carbohydrates that are recommended for the DASH Diet include green leafy vegetables, whole grains, low glycemic index fruits, legumes, beans, nuts, and seeds.

• Fats: Not all fats are created equally. Good fats can help maintain homeostasis in the body by preventing inflammation. Fats that are good for you are sourced from olive oil, avocadoes, nuts, flaxseed, hempseed, and fish's rich in Omega-3 fatty acids.

• Proteins: Similar to fats, not all proteins are created equally. The DASH Diet recommends more servings of plant-based proteins from legumes, nuts, and seeds. For animal protein, you can only consume lean meats, chicken, turkey, eggs, fish, and low-fat dairy.

Chapter 5   DASH Diet Food No-Goes

With the DASH Diet, nothing is technically off-limits, but dieters are recommended to eat less of foods that are bad for the health. But if you are new to this diet, it is crucial that you know about which foods you should avoid and which foods to avoid if you want to be successful in following the DASH Diet.

•   Red meat: Red meat is not recommended if you want to follow the DASH Diet. However, you can occasionally eat grass-fed beef as it is high in Omega-3 fatty acid due to its diet.

•   Bad fats: Not all fats are created equally. Avoid bad fats, including margarine, hydrogenated vegetable oil, and vegetable shortening, because they promote atherogenesis.

•   Salt or Sodium: The DASH Diet is a low salt diet or none at all as salt can cause hypertension. Instead of using salt, use the spice rack to improve the flavor of your food.

•   Alcohol: Consumption of alcohol can elevate your blood pressure levels. Too much alcohol can eventually damage the liver, brain, and heart. If you cannot avoid but drink alcohol, make sure that you drink one glass if you are a woman and two if you are a man.

•   Cured meats: All kinds of cured meats are not recommended because they contain high amounts of Sodium that may cause hypertension. Moreover, cured meats also contain potential carcinogens that can cause cancer.

- Full-fat dairy: The purpose of the DASH Diet is to lessen the intake of fat. This includes full-fat dairy, such as milk, cream, and cheese.

- Other foods: Other foods that are included in the no-eat list include high-fat snacks, sugary sweets or snacks, salad dressings, sauces, and gravies.

Low Sodium Philosophy

Sodium is the culprit of hypertension as it is widely known to increase blood pressure levels. Several studies have backed the dangers of consuming too much salt in your diet. When too much salt is taken in, it causes imbalance as well as reduce the ability of the body to regulate the excretion of fluid by the kidneys.

The American Heart Association released a dietary guideline on the amount of Sodium that an average American should take in. The average American takes in five or more teaspoons of salt daily, while the recommended daily allowance is 1,500 mg per day. This is like taking in 20 times as much as the body needs of salt every day.

It is vital to take note that Sodium is not only found in salt but also in many types of food so if you are not careful about the kinds of food you are going to eat, you are probably eating twice as much Sodium without even knowing it. Large amounts of Sodium are hidden in processed and canned foods. Your fast food favorites are also laden with Sodium. The thing is that if you are not careful with the food that you are eating, you may end up suffering from hypertension and other types of diseases.

The low Sodium philosophy encourages people to consume less salt by minding what they eat. Reading labels is very important so that you will know whether you are consuming too much salt on your food or not. Foods rich in Sodium are those labeled with brine, salt, and monosodium glutamate.

While the DASH Diet encourages people to cook meals from scratch using whole food ingredients, buying pre-packaged meals under this diet is highly unlikely. Under this philosophy, you are encouraged to eat more home-cooked meals because you know how much salt you are putting in your

food. But more than food, this particular philosophy also encourages people to avoid using medications that contain high amounts of Sodium, including Alka Seltzer and Bromo Seltzer. The thing is that anything that contains high amounts of Sodium – from food, beverage to medication – should be avoided when following the low Sodium philosophy.

Big Stride into the DASH Diet

DASH Diet Eating Guide

This section will serve as your guide on the types of food that you should eat to be successful while following the DASH Diet.

It is crucial to take note that the DASH Diet requires certain numbers of servings daily from different food groups. However, the number of calories needed by the body largely depends on how many calories you need daily. Moreover, it also depends on how well you have adjusted to this particular diet regimen. For instance, you can start with 2,400mg of Sodium daily first then you can gradually omit Sodium from salt eventually once you have gotten used to the diet eventually. Nevertheless, it is still essential that you know the general rules when it comes to planning your daily meals following the DASH Diet.

•   Add a serving of vegetables and fruits for both lunch and dinner. You can also eat fruits for snacking but make sure that they are not dried or canned because they have added sugar.

•   Use only half a serving of oil when cooking food.

•   Opt for low-fat dairy any time you would use full-fat dairy in cooking different recipes.

•   Limit your meat to only 6 ounces daily. It is advisable to make more vegetarian meals while following this diet. Proteins from animals should be substituted with beans or legumes.

•   Snack on unsalted chips, pretzels, or nuts. You can also opt for raw vegetables such as carrots and cucumber for snacks.

Now that you know the types of foods that you can eat following the DASH Diet, you need to know the number of different foods that you need to consume daily. Going back to the DASH Diet food pyramid, you can follow the suggested daily serving's specific to your caloric requirement. It is important to take note that the serving sizes of food in the DASH Diet is not what you are used to, compared with other eating plans. Below is an in-depth guide of the single serving sizes for each food groups listed above.

Table 1. Daily servings of food for people with varying caloric requirement and sample foods allowed in the DASH Diet

Food Group	1,600-calorie	2,000-calorie	1 serving equivalent
Grains (whole grains)	6 servings daily	6 to 8 servings daily	- 1 slice whole wheat bread - 1-ounce whole grain cereal - ½ cooked cereal, brown rice, or pasta (whole grain)
Vegetables	3 to 4 servings daily	4 to 5 servings daily	- 1 cup leafy green vegetables - ½ cup chopped raw or cooked vegetables - ½ cup low-sodium vegetable juice or broth
Fruits	4 servings daily	4 to 5 servings daily	- 1 medium-sized fruit - ¼ cup dried fruit - ½ cup fresh, frozen, or canned fruits

			- ½ cup 100% unsweetened fruit juice
Low-fat dairy	2 to 3 servings daily	2 to 3 servings daily	- 1 cup low-fat or fat-free milk - 1 cup low-fat or fat-free yogurt - 1 ½ ounces low-fat or fat-free cheese
Lean meats, poultry, and fish	3 to 4 ounces servings or less	6 ounces servings or less	- 1 egg - 2 egg whites - 1-ounce cooked lean meat, skinless
Nuts, seeds, and legumes	3 to 4 servings a week	4 to 5 servings a week	- 1/3 cup nuts (1 ½ ounces) - 2 tablespoons peanut butter - 2 tablespoons seeds (1/2 ounces) - ½ cup cooked legumes (dried beans)
Fats and oils	2 servings a day	2 to 3 servings a day	- 1 teaspoon soft margarine - 1 teaspoon vegetable oil - 1 tablespoon mayonnaise - 2 tablespoons low-fat salad dressing (1 tablespoon regular dressing)
Sweets and added	3 or fewer servings a week	5 or fewer servings a	- 1 tablespoon sugar - 1 tablespoon jam or jelly

sugar		week	- ½ cup sorbet, naturally sweetened
			- 1 cup sugar-sweetened lemonade

Chapter 6   Weight Maintenance Diet Patterns

Usually, though, the DASH diet attracts people because they have been diagnosed with high blood pressure and their doctor has advised them to seek out the kind of lifestyle changes that the DASH diet offers. Regardless of the reasons why you came to the DASH diet, it can lead to substantial weight loss.

The DASH diet really isn't all that difficult to follow, because in many cases it simply mirrors what people normally eat already, with just a few adjustments. So instead of eating barbecued pork ribs, you eat a skinless barbecued chicken breast. You can have potato salad but use low-fat mayo. Adjustments like these really aren't all that difficult. Compare that to following a keto or Atkins diet, where you can't consume either barbecue sauce or eat potatoes. If your friend is having a July 4th party, they may not invite the keto dieters.

Portion Control

Remember Weight Watchers? It is basically designed for portion control – but it uses a complicated system. Most people don't want to mix accounting with eating, so weight watchers may still attract a lot of adherents but most people don't want to bother with that.

Other diets which fall into the low-fat category are based largely on counting calories. These types of diets can leave you feeling hungry and irritable. You may grow tired and mentally foggy since your body isn't getting enough to get by and you're not feeling full.

The DASH diet avoids calorie counting altogether. Instead, you simply follow the rules for the portion sizes outlined earlier, and then eat the number of items that the DASH food pyramid advises, provided you're not overindulging.

By specifying the maximum number of portions you can eat each day from each food group, you automatically get portion control without having to count calories or follow some complicated system. With an emphasis on low-calorie fruits and veggies and the consumption of a lot of fiber, you will also find that you fill yourself up to more easily. That way you never feel deprived, even though you're limiting portion sizes and numbers of portions consumed daily.

Limited Meat Consumption

We aren't advocating that people become vegan or vegetarian, although that is an option if you want to pursue it. But if you don't, one benefit of following the DASH diet is that it limits meat consumption. Meat in and of itself is not necessarily a bad thing, but remember that meat is dense in calories. In American society, people eat meat without any regard to portion size or even how many times per day they are eating it. Many people eat some kind of meat item for breakfast, lunch, and dinner. They might even snack on it.

The DASH diet forces you to think about how much meat you're eating, maybe for the very first time in your life. It also restricts servings of meat to 0-2 servings per day. That's a very easy rule to follow, and if you are following it for the first time you're going to be reducing the overall level of calories consumed per day on a practically autopilot level.

By cutting out the fat on beef and pork and skin on poultry, another source of calories can be eliminated. This also contributes to weight loss if you haven't been paying much attention to that up until this moment.

Eat Those Fruits and Veggies

What's one of the top benefits of eating several servings of spinach? Well, it's packed with all kinds of cancer-fighting nutrients and contains important minerals like potassium, but the advantage we're looking for here is that spinach is very low calorie. So you can eat a lot of spinach, broccoli, cauliflower, and other veggies and fill your stomach up without even thinking about it. The high fiber content of fruits and vegetables will help you feel satiated faster and reduce the temptation to eat a lot of meats and oils. The result of this is more weight loss.

Regulating Sweets

The DASH diet will help you get a handle on sweets and desserts – provided that you're truly committed to the diet, of course. First, the DASH diet tells you exactly how many servings to eat – five per week. Second, it has strict definitions of what counts as a "sweet" with the size of each serving specified in detail. Sure – you could cheat if you wanted – but then don't blame anyone else if you fail to reach your health and weight loss goals. However, if you follow the rules you will find the fact that the DASH diet allows some sweets will help you satisfy that old sweet tooth and secondly that you will be losing weight despite consuming five servings of sweets per week.

The DASH diet does not make pie in the sky promises about weight loss. Keto, Atkins, and many other diets do make such claims. The DASH diet takes an entirely different approach, more akin to the turtle that wins the race rather than the hare, who has a good start in the race but loses.

The DASH diet, provided that you actually follow the rules, will generate slow but steady weight loss that will add up over time. Once you fully adjust to the rules to be followed on the diet you will find that it gets easier to follow as time goes on. When people get tired of avoiding pasta for the rest of their lives, and cheat on their deprivation diets you'll still be following yours since it's not much different from what people would eat already, it's just a healthier version of it with the relative proportions of foods changed around to promote more consumption of potassium and magnesium.

Simple Rules for Weight loss with Mediterranean Diet

There are various benefits this diet offers. If you really want to obtain all these benefits and maximize the returns on this diet, then there are a few rules you must follow. You will learn about the seven cardinal rules of the Mediterranean diet that will facilitate weight loss.

The rule about vegetables

There are a couple of dietary changes you need to make while following the Mediterranean diet. The first change is that you must increase your intake of vegetables. You must be wondering about the portion of vegetables you required to consume daily. Ensure that your intake of vegetables is about two to three cups daily. Include some form of vegetables or the other with every meal you consume.

The rule about meats

The Mediterranean diet is predominantly plant-based. Try avoiding or at least limiting your intake of red meat. Instead of consuming red meat twice or thrice a week, replace it with naturally fatty fish and other seafood. Don't think of meat as the major portion of a meal and start using it as a topping. For instance, you can add grilled meat to a salad instead of consuming steak. Make sure that every meal you consume is rich in vegetables instead of meats.

The rule about dairy products

Include some form of dairy products for all your meals. However, you must be mindful of your intake of milk. Greek yogurt, as well as cheese, is permitted with this diet. You can always add a little portion of cheese to your daily meals.

The rule about fruits

Start including plenty of fresh fruits to your daily meals. In fact, if you have a sweet tooth, go through the different Mediterranean diet-friendly desserts given in this book. Apart from this, you can also start consuming fruits to end your meals on a sweet note. Instead of sugar-rich processed foods, opt for seasonal fruits. You're free to consume plenty of fresh fruits!

The rule about fats

This diet encourages the consumption of healthy fats. Instead of any other cooking oil, start using olive oil and other nut-based butter. You don't have to worry about your intake of healthy fats. As long as you consume olive oil and avocado oil, it is all good.

The rule about grains

This diet doesn't place any restrictions on the consumption of grains. Only consume whole grains and stay away from processed flours. Whole grains are rich in nutrients, dietary fiber, and other vitamins that your body requires. Whole grains are also quite filling and low on the glycemic index.

The rule about processed foods

You must stay away from all sorts of processed foods. If anything looks like it was manufactured in a factory, avoid it. This applies to breakfast cereals, fruit juices, and any other food products you can think of. Whenever you shop for groceries, stay away from processed food aisle. Even those products that are labeled as low fat or diet are also not good for you. Always carefully read the labels before you purchase any products. Even processed meats must be avoided.

Chapter 7   Best Diet Tips to Lose Weight and Improve Health

Let's be honest — there's a mind-boggling measure of data on the Internet about how to immediately shed pounds and get fit as a fiddle.

If you're searching for the best tips on the most proficient method to get in shape and keep it off, this apparently interminable measure of counsel can be overpowering and confounding.

From the diets elevating crude foods to dinner designs that rotate around shakes and prepackaged foods, another prevailing fashion diet appears to spring up each day.

The issue is, albeit prohibitive diets and disposal feast plans will in all likelihood bring about transient weight loss, the vast majority can't keep up them and wind up quitting inside half a month.

Despite the fact that shedding 10 pounds (4.5 kg) in seven days by following a prevailing fashion diet may appear to be enticing, actually this sort of weight loss is often unhealthy and unsustainable.

The genuine key to sheltered and effective weight loss is to embrace a healthy lifestyle that suits your individual needs and that you can keep up forever.

The accompanying tips are healthy, practical approaches to get you in the groove again and headed towards your weight and wellness objectives.

Here are 25 of the best dieting tips to improve your health and assist you with getting more fit.

1. Top off on Fiber

Fiber is found in healthy foods including vegetables, organic products, beans and entire grains.

A few investigations have demonstrated that basically eating more fiber-rich foods may assist you with getting in shape and keep it off.

2. Jettison Added Sugar

Included sugar, particularly from sugary beverages, is a significant purpose behind unhealthy weight addition and health issues like diabetes and coronary illness.

Also, foods like treats, pop and prepared merchandise that contain heaps of added sugars will in general be low in the supplements your body needs to remain healthy.

Removing foods high in included sugars is an incredible method to lose overabundance weight.

It's imperative to take note of that even foods advanced as "healthy" or "natural" can be extremely high in sugar. Therefore, perusing nourishment marks is an absolute necessity.

3. Prepare for Healthy Fat

While fat is often the primary thing that gets slice when you're attempting to thin down, healthy fats can really assist you with arriving at your weight loss objectives.

Likewise, fats assist you with remaining more full for more, diminishing desires and helping you remain on track.

4. Limit Distractions

While expending dinners before your TV or PC may not appear as though diet harm, eating while diverted may make you devour more calories and put on weight.

Having during supper, away from potential interruptions, isn't just a decent method to hold your weight down — it likewise permits you an opportunity to reconnect with friends and family.

Cell phones are another gadget you should save while you're eating. Looking through messages or your Instagram or Facebook channel is similarly as diverting as a TV or PC.

5. Walk Your Way to Health

Numerous individuals accept they should receive a thorough exercise routine to kick off weight loss.

While different kinds of movement are significant when you're endeavoring to get fit as a fiddle, strolling is an astounding and simple approach to consume calories.

Actually, only 30 minutes of strolling every day has been appeared to help in weight loss.

Furthermore, it's an agreeable action that you can do both inside and outside whenever of day.

6. Draw out Your Inner Chef

Preparing more suppers at home has been appeared to advance weight loss and healthy eating.

Despite the fact that eating suppers at cafés is pleasant and can fit into a healthy diet plan, concentrating on preparing more dinners at home is an incredible method to hold your weight under tight restraints.

Furthermore, getting ready suppers at home enables you to explore different avenues regarding new, healthy fixings while setting aside you cash simultaneously.

7. Have a Protein-Rich Breakfast

Counting protein-rich foods like eggs in your morning meal has been appeared to profit weight loss.

Essentially swapping your everyday bowl of oat for a protein-pressed scramble made with eggs and sauteed veggies can assist you with shedding pounds.

Expanding protein consumption toward the beginning of the day may likewise assist you with staying away from unhealthy eating and improve hunger control for the duration of the day.

8. Try not to Drink Your Calories

While a great many people realize they ought to keep away from soft drinks and milkshakes, numerous individuals don't understand that even beverages publicized to support athletic execution or improve health can be stacked with undesirable fixings.

Sports drinks, espresso refreshments and enhanced waters will in general be extremely high in calories, artificial colorings and included sugar.

Indeed, even squeeze, which is often advanced as a healthy refreshment, can prompt weight gain if you devour excessively.

Concentrate on hydrating with water to limit the quantity of calories you drink for the duration of the day.

9. Shop Smart

Making a shopping rundown and adhering to it is an incredible method to abstain from purchasing unhealthy foods imprudently.

Also, making a shopping list has been appeared to prompt healthier eating and advance weight loss.

Another approach to restrict unhealthy buys at the market is to have a healthy supper or nibble before you go out to shop.

Studies have indicated that eager customers will in general reach for fattier, unhealthy foods.

10. Remain Hydrated

Drinking enough water for the duration of the day is useful for generally speaking health and can even assist you with keeping up a healthy weight.

One investigation of more than 9,500 individuals found that the individuals who were not enough hydrated had higher weight records (BMIs) and were bound to be hefty than the individuals who were appropriately hydrated (16).

Furthermore, individuals who drink water before suppers have been appeared to eat less calories.

11. Practice Mindful Eating

Hurrying through suppers or eating in a hurry may lead you to expend excessively, too rapidly.

Rather, be aware of your food, concentrating on how each nibble tastes. It might lead you to be increasingly mindful of when you are full, diminishing your odds of gorging (18).

Concentrating on eating gradually and making the most of your dinner, regardless of whether you have restricted time, is an extraordinary method to diminish gorging.

12. Cut Back on Refined Carbs

Refined carbs incorporate sugars and grains that have had their fiber and different supplements expelled. Models incorporate white flour, pasta and bread.

These sorts of foods are low in fiber, are processed rapidly and just keep you full for a brief timeframe.

Rather, pick wellsprings of complex sugars like oats, antiquated grains like quinoa and grain, or veggies like carrots and potatoes.

They'll help keep you more full for more and contain a lot a greater number of supplements than refined wellsprings of starches.

13. Lift Heavier to Get Lighter

Albeit high-impact practice like energetic strolling, running and biking is fantastic for weight loss, numerous individuals will in general spotlight exclusively on cardio and don't add quality preparing to their schedules.

Adding weight lifting to your exercise center routine can assist you with building more muscle and tone your whole body.

Likewise, thinks about have indicated that weight lifting gives your digestion a little lift, helping you consume more calories for the duration of the day, in any event, when you are very still (20).

14. Set Meaningful Goals

Fitting into pants from secondary school or glancing better in a bathing suit are famous reasons why individuals need to get thinner.

Nonetheless, it's significantly more important to genuinely comprehend why you need to get in shape and the manners in which that weight loss may decidedly influence your life. Having these objectives as a top priority may assist you with adhering to your arrangement.

Having the option to play tag with your kids or having the stamina to move throughout the night at a friend or family member's wedding are instances of objectives that can keep you focused on a positive change.

15. Maintain a strategic distance from Fad Diets

Prevailing fashion diets are elevated for their capacity to assist individuals with shedding pounds quick.

Nonetheless, these diets will in general be extremely prohibitive and difficult to keep up. This prompts yo-yo dieting, where individuals lose pounds, just to restore them.

While this cycle is basic in those attempting to take care of business rapidly, yo-yo dieting has been connected to a more noteworthy increment in body weight after some time.

Moreover, contemplates have demonstrated that yo-yo dieting can build the danger of diabetes, coronary illness, hypertension and metabolic disorder.

These diets might be enticing, however finding a practical, healthy eating plan that sustains your body as opposed to denying it is a vastly improved decision.

16. Eat Whole Foods

Monitoring precisely what is going into your body is an extraordinary method to get healthy.

Eating entire foods that don't accompany a fixing list guarantees that you are supporting your body with normal, supplement thick foods.

When buying foods with fixing records, toning it down would be ideal.

If an item has heaps of fixings that you are new to, odds are it isn't the healthiest choice.

17. Pal Up

If you are experiencing difficulty adhering to an exercise normal or healthy eating plan, welcome a companion to go along with you and assist you with remaining on track.

Studies show that individuals who thin down with a companion are bound to stay with weight loss and exercise programs. They additionally will in general lose more weight than the individuals who go only it.

In addition, having a companion or relative with a similar health and wellbeing objectives can assist you with remaining spurred while having a fabulous time simultaneously.

18. Try not to Deprive Yourself

Disclosing to yourself that you will never have your preferred foods again isn't just ridiculous, however it might likewise set you up for disappointment.

Denying yourself will just make you need the prohibited food more and may make you gorge when you at long last collapse.

Accounting for suitable extravagances to a great extent will show you poise and prevent you from feeling angry of your new, healthy lifestyle.

Having the option to appreciate a little segment of a custom made sweet or enjoying a most loved occasion dish is a piece of having a healthy association with food.

19. Be Realistic

Contrasting yourself with models in magazines or famous people on TV isn't just unreasonable — it can likewise be unhealthy.

While having a healthy good example can be an extraordinary method to remain propelled, being excessively condemning of yourself can interfere with you and may prompt unhealthy practices.

Give centering a shot how you feel as opposed to focusing on what you look like. Your fundamental inspirations ought to be to get more joyful, fitter and healthier.

20. Veg Out

Vegetables are stacked with fiber and the supplements your body hungers for.

In addition, expanding your vegetable admission can assist you with getting more fit.

Truth be told, ponders show that just eating a serving of mixed greens before a supper can assist you with feeling full, making you eat less.

Moreover, topping off on veggies for the duration of the day can assist you with keeping up a healthy weight and may diminish your danger of creating interminable sicknesses like coronary illness and diabetes

21. Bite Smart

Nibbling on unhealthy foods can cause weight gain.

A simple method to help shed pounds or keep up a healthy weight is to attempt to have healthy snacks accessible at home, in your vehicle and at your work environment.

For instance, reserving pre-distributed servings of blended nuts in your vehicle or having cut-up veggies and hummus prepared in your refrigerator can assist you with remaining on track when a hankering strikes.

22. Fill the Void

Fatigue may lead you to go after unhealthy foods.

Studies have indicated that being exhausted adds to an expansion in generally calorie utilization because it impacts individuals to eat more food, healthy and unhealthy.

Finding new exercises or side interests that you appreciate is a great method to abstain from gorging brought about by weariness.

Essentially taking a walk and getting a charge out of nature can help show signs of improvement attitude to remain persuaded and adhere to your health objectives.

23. Set aside a few minutes for yourself

Making a healthier lifestyle implies finding an opportunity to put yourself first, regardless of whether you don't believe it's conceivable.

Life often hinders weight loss and wellness objectives, so it is imperative to make an arrangement that incorporates individual time, and stick to it.

Obligations like work and child rearing are the absolute most significant things in life, however your health ought to be one of your top needs.

Regardless of whether that implies setting up a healthy lunch to bring to work, going for a run or going to a wellness class, putting aside time to deal with yourself can do ponders for both your physical and emotional wellness.

24. Discover Workouts You Actually Enjoy

The extraordinary thing about picking an exercise routine is that there are unlimited conceivable outcomes.

While perspiring through a turn class probably won't be some tea, mountain biking in a recreation center may be more suited to your abilities.

Certain exercises consume a larger number of calories than others. Be that as it may, you shouldn't pick an exercise dependent on the outcomes you think you'll get from it.

It's imperative to discover exercises that you anticipate doing and that satisfy you. That way you are bound to stay with them.

25. Backing Is Everything

Having a gathering of companions or relatives that supports you in your weight and wellbeing objectives is basic for effective weight loss.

Encircle yourself with constructive individuals who make you like making a healthy lifestyle will assist you with remaining spurred and on track.

Actually, thinks about have demonstrated that going to help gatherings and having a solid informal community assists individuals with getting in shape and keep it off (32).

Imparting your objectives to reliable and empowering loved ones can assist you with remaining responsible and set you up for progress.

If you don't have a strong family or gathering of companions, have a go at joining a care group. There are countless gatherings that meet face to face or on the web.

While there are numerous approaches to get in shape, finding a healthy eating and exercise plan that you can pursue for life is the most ideal approach to guarantee effective, long haul weight loss.

In spite of the fact that prevailing fashion diets may offer a convenient solution, they are often unhealthy and deny the body of the supplements and calories it needs, driving the vast majority to come back to unhealthy propensities after they hit their weight loss objective.

Being progressively dynamic, concentrating on entire foods, decreasing included sugar and setting aside a few minutes for yourself are only a couple of approaches to get healthier and more joyful.

Keep in mind, weight loss isn't one-size-fits-all. To be fruitful, it is essential to discover an arrangement that works for you and fits well with your lifestyle.

It is anything but a win or bust procedure, either. If you can't focus on every one of the recommendations in this book, take a stab at beginning with only a not many that you think will work for you. They'll assist you with arriving at your health and wellbeing objectives in a protected and reasonable manner.

Chapter 8   The DASH Diet and
Hypertension/High Blood Pressure

In the United States, it's estimated that about 50 million people are suffering from high blood pressure. The actual number is unknown, and it's often called "the silent killer". The reason is that someone can appear to be completely healthy and yet have high blood pressure.

In many cases, high blood pressure can be due to family history or genetics. However many environmental causes exist as well, and even if you have a family history your lifestyle choices may work against you or for you, however, the case may be. In other words, you might have the family history but if you don't smoke, maintain your weight, and exercise, you might avoid developing high blood pressure. Conversely, maybe you're relatively healthy even though you have a family history. Adopting an unhealthy lifestyle habit like smoking might tip you over the edge, leading to hypertension.

Some of the most common causes that have been identified include:

- Smoking: Cigarette smoking in particular, due to the fact people get more nicotine in their system, has been strongly identified as an environmental risk factor for developing high blood pressure.

- Weight gain/obesity: Not all overweight people have high blood pressure, but it's clear that being overweight significantly increases your risk of developing it. The heavier you get the higher the risk.

- Sedentary lifestyle: Exercise definitely counteracts hypertension. It helps keep the blood vessels flexible and responsive and helps keep the heart in shape. Someone who has cardiovascular fitness has a lower resting heart rate and their heart pumps with a healthier level of force, so the blood pressure is reduced as compared to what it would be otherwise. In contrast, people who don't exercise raise their risk of developing high blood pressure, especially if they have a family history.

- Race: African Americans are more prone to high blood pressure than other groups. However, bear in mind that all racial and ethnic groups have plenty of risk of high blood pressure and its victims include people of all races and from every country across the globe.

- Kidney disease: The kidneys are closely tied to the healthy maintenance of blood sugar. They help regulate the amount of fluid and salt in the body. When you are suffering from kidney disease they may not function as well, and this may lead to fluid and sodium retention which can cause high blood pressure.

- Age: Simply getting older raises risk, although we would never call high blood pressure "normal". However, as you get older things don't work as well (you knew that, right?). If your joints are stiffening you can bet your arteries are as well. So even though you may be reasonably healthy overall, simply getting older raises your risk of developing some level of high blood pressure. There is some debate about whether older people need to be put under the same standards as to what constitutes a diagnosis of hypertension or not, but a general rule applies. You're better off if your blood pressure is below 140/100.

- Nutritional deficiencies: By now you're an expert – nutritional deficiencies of potassium and magnesium can lead to the development of high blood pressure, along with other health problems like heart palpitations and muscle cramps.

- Excessive salt in the diet: We've reviewed this one already – salt causes your body to retain fluid and it promotes contraction of blood vessels, among other things.

The DASH diet provides an opportunity to address several items on this list. It reduces salt in the diet and addresses the nutritional deficiencies in potassium and magnesium. By consuming large amounts of fruits and vegetables along with a low-fat diet, you'll find that your risk of kidney disease drops as well. Controlling weight can also reduce the risks of developing high blood pressure.

What is Metabolic Syndrome?

We now turn our attention to one of the biggest health problems of the age: *metabolic syndrome*. In many cases, people who have high blood pressure are actually suffering from metabolic syndrome, and by following the DASH diet, they won't just cure their high blood pressure, they will reset their metabolism and eliminate metabolic syndrome from their lives.

Aside: Your Blood Lipids

Before we formally define metabolic syndrome, we need to review some basics about blood chemistry. The first area we need to review are blood lipids, which are basically the fats flowing around in your blood. Kind of gross, huh?

Don't worry, it's all perfectly natural and you need some level of blood fats. These fats take on a few different forms, some in combination with other molecules. This isn't a chemistry class so we aren't going to concern ourselves with the gory details, but we need to know what is in your blood and what the healthy levels of various components should be. Generally, we are concerned with the following:

- Total cholesterol

- LDL cholesterol

- HDL cholesterol

- Triglycerides

No doubt you've heard about total cholesterol already, it's been the focus of the medical community for many years. High total cholesterol is associated with increased risk of developing heart disease, and also with a higher risk of actually having a heart attack or stroke. In the United States, we measure cholesterol in milligrams of cholesterol per deciliter of blood, or mg/dL. A general rule of thumb is that a total cholesterol of 200 or less is considered low risk, while total cholesterol over 200 is considered elevated risk, with the risk significantly increasing for each 10 point increase in your total cholesterol. If you consistently show total cholesterol levels of 230 mg/dL or higher, your doctor may want to prescribe statin drugs, which lower cholesterol. Some doctors are more strict than others and will prescribe statins at even lower levels.

Total cholesterol is calculated the following way:

Total cholesterol = LDL Cholesterol + HDL Cholesterol + 0.20 * Triglycerides

You will often see your triglyceride level shown on your blood tests, what this means is that 20% of your triglyceride level is counted toward your total cholesterol number. Triglycerides are a type of fat that is carried around in your blood.

LDL means Low-Density Lipoprotein. A lipoprotein is a complicated molecule that is made of fat ("lipo") and proteins. Cholesterol is actually a substance transported through the blood by the LDL or HDL molecule.

LDL is called "bad cholesterol" because it can stick to the walls of your arteries. Over time, they become calcified and you develop fatty deposits and plaque, and the arteries can narrow, eventually causing a heart attack. The level of LDL cholesterol in your blood is directly related to the amount of saturated fat you eat per day. An easy way to lower your cholesterol if you're in the borderline range and your doctor isn't putting you on statins yet is to limit your consumption of saturated fats to 20 grams per day or less. Saturated fat is mostly found in animal products like beef and chicken skin, but it's in all animal products. Dairy and even fish also contain saturated fat. Coconut oil also contains a lot of saturated fat.

HDL is known as "good cholesterol". The reason is that HDL cholesterol is sort of a cleanup crew for the bloodstream. It picks up bad cholesterol, even cleaning it off the artery walls, and it brings it back to the liver. If you have a higher HDL cholesterol (greater than 45 mg/dL, about) then you're at lower risk of heart disease.

The ratio of total cholesterol to HDL can predict your risk of a heart attack. Generally, you're at lower risk of heart attack if:

Total Cholesterol/HDL < 5

So if someone has total cholesterol of 200 and an HDL cholesterol of 50, their ratio is:

200/50 = 4

This person is considered at low risk of having a heart attack over say, the next five years. Now suppose someone had total cholesterol of 220 and an HDL cholesterol of 35. Their ratio would be:

220/35 = 6.3

This person is at elevated risk for a heart attack. Their physician may put them on a statin and advise them to take up vigorous aerobic exercise.

While a ratio of less than five is desirable, a ratio of about 3 is considered ideal. While lowering total cholesterol can be achieved with statins, it's not really possible to raise HDL with any drugs. A better diet, losing weight, and exercise may raise your HDL.

Although cholesterol is portrayed as some kind of dangerous substance, it's actually a key component of the body. It's used to build and maintain cell membranes, and it's used to make important hormones in the body. You'd die without any cholesterol, and in fact, people with very low cholesterol (below 160) have higher rates of death from all causes.

Triglycerides are also important to measure. High triglycerides indicate a higher risk of heart attack and can cause other problems such as pancreatitis. The ratio of triglycerides to HDL cholesterol is a good indicator of heart attack risk, in fact, it's better than looking at total cholesterol or even LDL "bad" cholesterol. If the ratio is 1 or less, you're considered to be at low risk of a heart attack. If it's greater than 1, then you're at higher risk.

High LDL cholesterol and a high triglyceride to HDL number not only indicate the risk of heart attack, but they are also a good way to evaluate the risk of stroke. To summarize, it's bad to have:

- High LDL cholesterol

- Low HDL cholesterol

- High triglycerides

Blood Sugar and Insulin

Now we move on from fat to sugar. Like cholesterol, your body needs some sugar in the blood. Without sugar, your brain can't power itself. And just like with cholesterol when your blood sugar goes too high, serious health problems will result.

The hormone insulin is closely tied to blood sugar. Basically, when you eat something your body begins to digest the carbohydrates in the food you ate. They are broken down into individual components called glucose, the simplest form of sugar or starch that there is. The glucose then enters your bloodstream.

The cells of your body need glucose for energy and your brain needs it to survive. However, the cells of the body aren't just going to suck up the glucose. They need a trigger, to be told to take it up. That trigger is provided by insulin. Think of insulin as a key fitting into the door of the cell and opening it, so that the glucose can go inside, and leave the bloodstream.

In a normal, healthy person, this process works fine. A healthy person could eat a plate of spaghetti, and about two hours later their blood sugar would be about 140 mg/dL (we measure blood sugar in the same units used to measure cholesterol).

However, some people begin to become resistant to insulin. Maybe you could think of it as the keys to the door wearing out, but over time, it takes more insulin to trigger the cells into taking up the sugar. The cells are said to become *insulin resistant.* As a result, the person is not getting the proper energy they need from the food, and their blood sugar goes higher than it does for a normal person after a meal. Eating that same plate of spaghetti, their blood sugar may go up to 180 mg/dL, or even 200 mg/dL. Blood sugar may stay elevated for longer periods of time. Eventually, the person will see blood sugar elevated even when fasting overnight. This is often the first sign that is caught by doctors that a patient may be pre-diabetic or diabetic.

The body isn't designed for elevated levels of glucose in the blood. High blood sugar will damage blood vessels, in particular, smaller blood vessels that supply organs and nerves. With reduced blood supply, over time various organs and nerves become damaged. This can cause kidney disease, vision problems, erectile dysfunction, and problems healing since the blood supply to peripheral wounds is compromised.

The pancreas, the organ that produces insulin, also suffers over time when someone has high blood sugars. In an attempt to compensate, it strains itself making more and more insulin. These things go together:

- A person who has high blood sugar
- Also has high levels of insulin
- And is insulin resistant

High glucose levels in the blood also damage your arteries. This leads to "hardening" of the arteries or atherosclerosis, which can lead to heart attack and stroke.

In addition, cancer cells love sugar. High blood sugar is associated with higher risks of cancer. In fact, diabetics have the higher risk for cancer as versus everyone else. Moreover, diabetics treated with the blood sugar controlling drug Metformin actually have a reduced risk of developing cancer.

Finally – Metabolic Syndrome

A person that has all these problems is said to have metabolic syndrome because the cluster of health problems are related to a dysfunctional metabolic system that is related to problems digesting simple carbohydrates.

A diagnosis of metabolic syndrome involves having three or more of the following:

- Increased weight around the midsection.

- Elevated blood sugar and insulin resistance.

- High total cholesterol.

- High triglycerides.

- Low HDL cholesterol

- High blood pressure, above 135/85.

So now we've tried everything together – the problems that we've been describing, including high blood pressure, low HDL cholesterol and elevated blood sugars, seldom occur in isolation. If you look at the symptoms, it kind of looks like middle age in developed countries, especially in the United States. There is no question it's related to the unhealthy eating practices of the standard American diet.

The DASH Diet and Metabolic Syndrome

The DASH diet is a good diet for tackling metabolic syndrome. The diet is also designed to reduce blood pressure levels. Moreover, the moderate level of consumption of lean meats will help lower total cholesterol. Since over time, it will also lead to weight loss, the DASH diet will create a feedback loop that will lead to further improvement in all of these measures. In short, the DASH diet is made to order for metabolic syndrome. If the characteristics of metabolic syndrome sounds like you at all – then you should be considering the DASH diet among your options.

Chapter 9   Your DASH Diet Primer

The DASH diet represents a balanced, varied style of eating that offers you a practical nutrition solution to help you move toward your goals. Healthy eating is complicated by all of the fad diets and trends in the world. We are going to ignore that and focus on a style of eating that you can really feel confident in. Here, we will take a closer look at why the DASH diet is so different, and so much better, than what you may be used to.

From the Standard American Diet to the DASH Diet

The average American's diet needs some improvement. Health concerns such as obesity, diabetes, and hypertension have become more of a norm than an exception. According to the 2013–2014 data from the National Health and Nutrition Examination Survey, more than two-thirds of the American population was considered either overweight or obese. This is partially due to a disconnect between the amount of calories we consume from food, the amount our bodies need, and the amount we expend through physical activity. What's much more concerning is the reality that approximately one in three American adults has high blood pressure, also known as hypertension, which is one of the most significant risk factors for cardiovascular disease. This does not even mention the fact that so few of us consume adequate amounts of the most healthful foods like fruits and vegetables.

This is where the Dietary Approaches to Stop Hypertension (DASH) eating style, which was developed and tested specifically with the purpose of addressing the pervasive issue of high blood pressure, or hypertension, comes in. First unveiled in an article in *The New England Journal of Medicine* in 1997, the DASH diet has grown in mainstream popularity, and was ranked as the number one Best Diet for Healthy Eating by the *U.S. News & World Report* in 2018, which also ranked it number four on the list of easiest diets to follow.

How DASH Diet Aids in Weight Loss and Lowers Blood Pressure

The DASH diet is highlighted by its inclusion of ample fruits, vegetables, and low-fat dairy products while also being generally low in saturated fat. The blood pressure lowering qualities of the DASH diet are often attributed to it being naturally high in potassium, calcium, and magnesium, which are found abundantly in the diverse array of foods that the diet incorporates.

In 2001, the DASH group conducted a follow-up study to the one published in 1997 and again published their results in *The New England Journal of Medicine*. The study found the DASH diet was even more effective at lowering blood pressure when combined with dietary sodium restriction. Excessive sodium, or salt, intake has since become well known to increase some people's risk for hypertension. Changes to diet while also restricting sodium has become recognized as effective to lower blood pressure. These DASH diet trials, and a number of others that followed, effectively proved that the DASH diet can significantly reduce your blood pressure.

But how does the DASH dietary pattern stack up for those who may be trying to lose weight? From my perspective as a registered dietitian, the DASH diet offers you the opportunity to shed unwanted pounds in a practical and nonrestrictive way. For example, the DASH diet contains plenty of fruits and whole grains, which many common diets restrict. It focuses on balanced and moderate inclusion of all different types of foods. With that in mind, it comes as no surprise that a 2016 review study published in the *Obesity Reviews* journal concluded that the "DASH diet is a good choice for weight management, particularly for weight reduction in overweight and obese participants."

Caloric Intake on the DASH Diet

The DASH diet guidelines center on the inclusion of a wide variety of food groups in amounts that vary based on individual characteristics. These food groups and their recommended serving sizes are determined by personal characteristics including your age, gender, and activity level. Before you can determine your own personal DASH diet guidelines, you need to estimate your calorie needs. The first two tables below will help you estimate your body's daily caloric needs. In order to figure out your estimated daily calorie intake, take a look at your physical activity. **Sedentary** is defined as little to no physical activity, **moderately active** as walking 1½ to 3 miles a day plus light physical activity, and **active** as exercising at the level suggested by the 28-day plan that follows.

Estimated Daily Calorie Needs for Women

AGE (YEARS)	SEDENTARY	MODERATELY ACTIVE	ACTIVE
19–30	2,000	2,100	2,400
31–50	1,800	2,000	2,200
51+	1,600	1,800	2,100

Estimated Daily Calorie Needs for Men

AGE (YEARS)	SEDENTARY	MODERATELY ACTIVE	ACTIVE
19–30	2,400	2,700	3,000
31–50	2,200	2,500	2,900
51+	2,000	2,300	2,600

Keep in mind that if your goal is to reduce your body weight, a simple first step is to consume approximately 250 to 500 calories fewer than what the above tables estimate. Please consult the charts below, which you can then use with the Daily Serving Recommendations table to determine your approximate serving recommendations for each food group. With that in mind, I want you to worry less about the actual number of calories you are aiming for and more about what this means in terms of total daily servings in the DASH diet.

Estimated Daily Calorie Needs for Women Who Want to Lose Weight

AGE (YEARS)	SEDENTARY	MODERATELY ACTIVE	ACTIVE
19–30	1,500–1,750	1,600–1,850	1,900–2,150
31–50	1,300–1,550	1,500–1,750	1,700–1,950
51+	1,100–1,350	1,300–1,550	1,600–1,850

Estimated Daily Calorie Needs for Men Who Want to Lose Weight

AGE (YEARS)	SEDENTARY	MODERATELY ACTIVE	ACTIVE
19–30	1,900-2,150	2,200–2,450	2,500–2,750
31–50	1,700-1,950	2,000–2,250	2,400–2,650
51+	1,500-1,750	1,800–2,050	2,100–2,350

The DASH Diet Guidelines

It is important to identify the different kinds of foods that the DASH diet encourages you to consume. There are some general guidelines to eating in a DASH-friendly way. You should limit the amount of sodium, sweets, sugary drinks, and red meat that you consume. But how and why? Let's discuss the different kinds of foods you should be consuming and why they help improve your health.

WHOLE GRAINS AND STARCHY VEGETABLES

Let's face it: Almost all of us love carbohydrate-rich foods, and although very-low-carb diets may help some lose weight in the short term, they aren't particularly sustainable and certainly not very enjoyable. The DASH diet doesn't suggest avoiding carbs; it suggests you enjoy the most fiber- and nutrient-dense versions of them, which is a message I can certainly get behind. Brown rice, quinoa, whole-grain bread, whole-grain pasta, and potatoes (any variety) are DASH-approved.

Serving size: 1 slice whole-grain bread, ½ cup brown rice or quinoa, 1 medium-size potato or sweet potato.

VEGETABLES

Vegetables are, simply put, the most important part of any eating style. The high potassium content of most vegetables—especially leafy greens—plays an important role in blood pressure regulation. Your kidneys play an important role in blood pressure management by controlling the fluid balance in your body. This balance is further modified by your sodium and potassium intake. Most people consume much more sodium than potassium, which affects your kidneys' ability to properly control your blood pressure. This balance can be restored in most people by increasing potassium intake and decreasing sodium intake. Vegetables contain a vast amount of other healthful nutrients and antioxidant compounds. From a weight-management perspective, the high fiber content of vegetables promotes satiety and may prevent weight gain. A 2009 study in *The Journal of Nutrition* found that women who increased their fiber intake tended to gain less weight and body fat over time. Most Americans simply do not eat enough fiber, with only about half the population consuming the American Heart Association's recommended daily target goal of 30 grams per day.

Serving size: ½ cup cooked veggies like broccoli or Brussels sprouts, 1 cup raw vegetables like spinach.

FRUIT

Sometimes popular "diets" suggest eliminating fruit because it contains moderate amounts of natural sugars. If this is something you've heard, I want you to ignore that sentiment and embrace fruit as a very healthy component of the DASH diet and a critical part of longevity and good health. Fruit, aside from being absolutely delicious, is rich in potassium, fiber, and other important nutrients that help support both blood pressure and weight management.

Serving size: 1 medium-size piece of fruit like an apple or banana, ½ cup fruit like blueberries or strawberries.

LOW-FAT DAIRY AND ALTERNATIVES

Dairy products and alternatives are an important part of the DASH eating plan for a few reasons. The high calcium content of these foods is thought to play an important role in blood-pressure regulation because it modifies the hormones that are responsible for the tension in your blood vessels. The high protein content also supports weight management and weight loss, because protein not only makes us feel full but requires extra energy for our bodies to break down. This largely explains why studies, including a 2015 review published in *The American Journal of Clinical Nutrition*, tend to find that adequate protein intake is usually associated with better outcomes when it comes to managing both our weight and our appetite.

Serving size: 1 cup skim milk, 1 cup 0% yogurt (including Greek), 1 cup soy milk, 1½ ounces skim cheese.

LEAN MEAT, POULTRY, FISH, AND ALTERNATIVES

These are dietary staples for many and important contributors of protein and magnesium in the DASH diet. For anyone who happens to be vegan or vegetarian, know that you can confidently replace animal-protein sources listed here with legume-based protein such as tofu, lentils, chickpeas, and others. When selecting meat, leaner cuts like tenderloin, sirloin, or eye of round for beef are optimal as they contain less fat than other commonly available varieties. Avoiding purchasing cuts with visible fat or trimming fat before cooking also helps. We suggest consuming multiple servings of fish per week.

Serving size: 1 ounce of cooked meat, poultry, or fish, 1 egg, 3 ounces of tofu

NUTS, SEEDS, AND LEGUMES

This group of foods is unique for the simple fact they are among the relatively small group of plant-based foods that contain both iron and protein, which are two of the important nutrients animal proteins offer us. Unlike most types of meat, though, these choices are high in fiber and heart-healthy monounsaturated fat while also being much lower in saturated fat.

Serving size: ⅓ cup raw or unsalted nuts or seeds, 2 tablespoons nut butter, ½ cup cooked legumes (preferably cooked from raw, not canned, which are higher in sodium).

HEALTHY FATS AND OILS

This group contains the types of foods we might either top food with or use to cook with. When people think of healthy fats, they often think about olive oil and other vegetable oils, which are a great choice and certainly better choices than the likes of lard or butter. Even so, it's important to be mindful of how much of these items we use because, in addition to being calorie-dense, many of the nutritional benefits of oils are offered in greater supply in foods like nuts and seeds, which also keep us feeling full due to their fiber content. We suggest making your own salad dressing out of oil and vinegar. If choosing store-bought, opt for the refrigerated versions, and be sure to read the labels and choose the lowest sodium version. We also offer salad dressing recipes that are better for you in our recipe section.

Serving size: 1 teaspoon oil, 2 tablespoons light salad dressing, 1 tablespoon standard dressing.

MORE ON OILS FROM CHEF JULIE

We want the majority of our fat intake from oils to come from unsaturated fats while a little can come from saturated. It is recommended to avoid trans fats, also known as hydrogenated oils. Depending on the type of fatty acids in oils and how they were processed, each has a unique smoke point or burn point, meaning different oils should be used for different applications.

•When cooking with high heat, such as roasting, stir-frying, or grilling, use neutral unsaturated oils, such as canola or avocado oil. Canola is relatively inexpensive yet contains omega-3 fatty acids. Avocado is also a great choice, as it's primarily made up of monounsaturated fatty acids and has the highest smoke point of all oils, but it's also a bit more expensive. They are both excellent cooking oils; it just depends on your personal choice and budget. For most of the recipes in this book, these oils are appropriate. I put "canola oil" in the recipes because it is the least expensive option, but feel free to use whichever one you prefer. If you are trying to avoid genetically modified organisms (GMOs), choose organic canola oil, as any food item that is labeled organic has to also be free of GMOs by law.

•When cooking with low heat, such as a quick sauté, or when making most salad dressings, use extra-virgin olive oil, which is also high in monounsaturated fats. It has a low smoke point, so it's best not to roast, stir-fry, or grill with it at high temperatures.

When an oil starts to burn, the chemical composition changes, and it may no longer be a healthy option. Other olive oils, like extra light, have been processed differently and have a higher smoke point. These are also great oils to use in higher-heat cooking if you prefer the olive oil flavor. I enjoy using olive oils for recipes that are Mediterranean-style, as the flavor lends itself well to those dishes.

There are many other oils on the market, and the ones I've mentioned above aren't the only nutritious options. We've chosen a handful of oils we regularly use because of their nutritional properties and cooking applications and have shared them with you to keep things simple and affordable.

Due to its recent popularity, we should also discuss coconut oil. The studies on it are mixed, given that it's a saturated fat but also a plant, so we generally recommend consuming it occasionally, such as when making a granola bar recipe or when baking.

SWEETS

The final proof that the DASH diet is quite unlike any diet you've probably tried before is that you can have dessert. Yes, you can have sweets, and—yes —you can have them more than just once a week. The unfortunate reality is that for many people, diets are difficult to maintain because of their restrictive nature. The DASH plan is a long-term sustainable eating style that promotes enjoying both food and life. Don't worry, you can still have ice cream in moderation.

Serving size: ½ cup ice cream or frozen yogurt; 1 tablespoon syrup, honey, or sugar; 1 cup juice or other sugar-sweetened drink.

SODIUM

Sodium, which is commonly known as the salt we find in or add to food, is often over consumed and one of the key drivers of high blood pressure. Specific strategies on how to consume sodium within the 2,300-milligram daily limit will be discussed at length below.

Goal: Under 2,300 milligrams daily to start (1 teaspoon), working toward a maximum 1,500 milligrams (¾ teaspoon) daily.

LOWER-SODIUM LIVING

In some people, prolonged excessive sodium intake contributes to high blood pressure partially because it can lead to chronic fluid retention, which ultimately strains your blood vessels. However, cutting the amount of salt in your diet may not be as simple as just putting away the shaker. It will, in fact, take a multifaceted approach for most people to make a significant dent in their daily intake. Let's take a closer look at the three areas where you can do this most effectively:

At the grocery store: Your mission to reduce the amount of sodium in your diet starts at the grocery store. Any food product sold in a box or a bottle, ranging from crackers to pasta sauces, could potentially have a very high sodium content. Your best defense is utilizing the labels on these products to compare sodium content among similar foods in the same category. Choosing the product that is lowest in sodium is a great first step.

At home: Did you know that a single teaspoon of salt contains your DASH diet sodium limit (2,300 milligrams) for the day? Those who don't add salt to their food won't be concerned by this, but if you are a heavy user it may be time to consider relying on herbs, spices, or sodium-free blends of both. When you use them in combination with acidic flavors such as those offered by lemon juice or vinegar, you won't miss a thing from a taste perspective and will ultimately need to rely less on sodium-heavy condiments from the grocery store.

Eating out: Any given meal purchased out, as compared to made at home, is likely to have significantly higher sodium content. This is problematic for those living with high blood pressure and especially true of selections that are heavy in sauces, such as pasta dishes. Other heavily salted restaurant items might include French fries or various soup dishes. For this reason, setting goals around how many meals you purchase out a week is an important part of your lifestyle going forward.

Chapter 10   Breakfast Recipes

1. Sunny-Side up Baked Eggs with Swiss chard, Feta, and Basil

Preparation time: 15 minutes

Cooking time: 10 to 15 minutes

Servings 4

Ingredients: GF NF 30 - 1 tablespoon extra-virgin olive oil, divided - ½ red onion, diced

½ teaspoon kosher salt - ¼ teaspoon nutmeg - ⅛ teaspoon freshly ground black pepper

4 cups Swiss chard, chopped - ¼ cup crumbled feta cheese - 4 large eggs

¼ cup fresh basil, chopped or cut into ribbons

Directions:

Preheat the oven to 375°F. Place 4 ramekins on a half sheet pan or in a baking dish and grease lightly with olive oil.

Heat the remaining olive oil in a large skillet or sauté pan over medium heat. Add the onion, salt, nutmeg, and pepper and sauté until translucent, about 3 minutes. Add the chard and cook, stirring, until wilted, about 2 minutes.

Split the mixture among the 4 ramekins. Add 1 tablespoon feta cheese to each ramekin. Crack 1 egg on top of the mixture in each ramekin. Bake for 10 to 12 minutes, or until the egg white is set.

Allow to cool for 1 to 2 minutes, then carefully transfer the eggs from the ramekins to a plate with a fork or spatula. Garnish with the basil.

Cooking tip: If you leave the eggs in the ramekins after removing them from the oven, they will continue to cook. If you want to serve the eggs in the ramekins, pull them from the oven a little early (after 8 to 10 minutes) so the yolks do not overcook.

Nutrition: Calories: 140 Total fat: 10g Sodium: 370mg Total Carbohydrates: 4g Protein: 9g

2. Harissa Shakshuka with Bell Peppers and Tomatoes

Preparation time: 10 minutes

Cooking time: 20 minutes

Servings 4

Ingredients: DF FF GF NF 1P 30 - 1½ tablespoons extra-virgin olive oil

2 tablespoons harissa - 1 tablespoon tomato paste - ½ onion, diced

1 bell pepper, seeded and diced - 3 garlic cloves, minced

1 (28-ounce) can no-salt-added diced tomatoes - ½ teaspoon kosher salt

4 large eggs - 2 to 3 tablespoons fresh basil, chopped or cut into ribbons

Directions:

Preheat the oven to 375°F.

Heat the olive oil in a 12-inch cast-iron pan or ovenproof skillet over medium heat. Add the harissa, tomato paste, onion, and bell pepper; sauté for 3 to 4 minutes. Add the garlic and cook until fragrant, about 30 seconds. Add the diced tomatoes and salt and simmer for about 10 minutes.

Make 4 wells in the sauce and gently break 1 egg into each. Transfer to the oven and bake until the whites are cooked and the yolks are set, 10 to 12 minutes.

Allow to cool for 3 to 5 minutes, garnish with the basil, and carefully spoon onto plates.

Nutrition:

Calories: 190

Total fat: 10g

Sodium: 255mg

Total Carbohydrates: 15g

Protein: 9g

3. Egg in a "Pepper Hole" with Avocado

Preparation time: 15 minutes

Cooking time: 5 minutes

Servings 4

Ingredients: DF FF GF NF 30 - 4 bell peppers, any color - 1 tablespoon extra-virgin olive oil

8 large eggs - ¾ teaspoon kosher salt, divided - ¼ teaspoon freshly ground black pepper, divided

1 avocado, peeled, pitted, and diced - ¼ cup red onion, diced

¼ cup fresh basil, chopped

Juice of ½ lime

Directions:

Stem and seed the bell peppers. Cut 2 (2-inch-thick) rings from each pepper. Chop the remaining bell pepper into small dice, and set aside.

Heat the olive oil in a large skillet over medium heat. Add 4 bell pepper rings, then crack 1 egg in the middle of each ring. Season with ¼ teaspoon of the salt and ⅛ teaspoon of the black pepper. Cook until the egg whites are mostly set but the yolks are still runny, 2 to 3 minutes. Gently flip and cook 1 additional minute for over easy. Move the egg–bell pepper rings to a platter or onto plates, and repeat with the remaining 4 bell pepper rings.

In a medium bowl, combine the avocado, onion, basil, lime juice, reserved diced bell pepper, the remaining ¼ teaspoon kosher salt, and the remaining ⅛ teaspoon black pepper. Divide among the 4 plates.

Nutrition: Calories: 270

Total fat: 19g

Sodium: 360mg

Total Carbohydrates: 12g

Fiber: 5g;

Sugars: 6g
Protein: 15g

4. Polenta with Sautéed Chard and Fried Eggs

Preparation time: 5 minutes

Cooking time: 20 minutes

Servings 4

Ingredients:GF NF 30

For the polenta - 2½ cups water - ½ teaspoon kosher salt - ¾ cups whole-grain cornmeal

¼ teaspoon freshly ground black pepper - 2 tablespoons grated Parmesan cheese

For the chard

1 tablespoon extra-virgin olive oil

1 bunch (about 6 ounces) Swiss chard, leaves and stems chopped and separated

2 garlic cloves, sliced - ¼ teaspoon kosher salt - ⅛ teaspoon freshly ground black pepper

Lemon juice (optional)

For the eggs - 1 tablespoon extra-virgin olive oil - 4 large eggs

Directions: To make the polenta

Bring the water and salt to a boil in a medium saucepan over high heat. Slowly add the cornmeal, whisking constantly. Decrease the heat to low, cover, and cook for 10 to 15 minutes, stirring often to avoid lumps. Stir in the pepper and Parmesan, and divide among 4 bowls.

To make the chard

Heat the oil in a large skillet over medium heat. Add the chard stems, garlic, salt, and pepper; sauté for 2 minutes. Add the chard leaves and cook until wilted, about 3 to 5 minutes.Add a spritz of lemon juice (if desired), toss together, and divide evenly on top of the polenta.

To make the eggs

Heat the oil in the same large skillet over medium-high heat. Crack each egg into the skillet, taking care not to crowd the skillet and leaving space between the eggs. Cook until the whites are set and golden around the edges, about 2 to 3 minutes.

Serve sunny-side up or flip the eggs over carefully and cook 1 minute longer for over easy. Place one egg on top of the polenta and chard in each bowl.Substitution tip: Any greens you like or have on hand will work well in this recipe.

Nutrition: Calories: 310 Total fat: 18g Sodium: 500mg Total Carbohydrates: 21g Protein: 17g

5. Smoked Salmon Egg Scramble with Dill and Chives

Preparation time: 5 minutes

Cooking time: 5 minutes

Servings 2

Ingredients:

FF GF NF 1P 30

4 large eggs

1 tablespoon milk

1 tablespoon fresh chives, minced

1 tablespoon fresh dill, minced

¼ teaspoon kosher salt

⅛ teaspoon freshly ground black pepper

2 teaspoons extra-virgin olive oil

2 ounces smoked salmon, thinly sliced

Directions:

In a large bowl, whisk together the eggs, milk, chives, dill, salt, and pepper.

Heat the olive oil in a medium skillet or sauté pan over medium heat. Add the egg mixture and cook for about 3 minutes, stirring occasionally.

Add the salmon and cook until the eggs are set but moist, about 1 minute.

Nutrition: Calories: 325

Total fat: 26g

Sodium: 455mg

Total Carbohydrates: 1g

Fiber: 0g

Protein: 23g

6. Berry Quinoa Bowls

Preparation Time: 35 Minutes

Cooking Time: 35 Minutes

Servings: 2

Ingredients:

1 Small Peach, Sliced

2/3 + ¾ Cup Milk, Low Fat

1/3 Cup Uncooked Quinoa, Rinsed Well

½ Teaspoon Vanilla Extract, Pure

2 Teaspoons Brown Sugar

14 Blueberries

2 Teaspoons Honey, Raw

12 Raspberries

Directions:

Start to boil your quinoa, vanilla, 2/3 cup milk and brown sugar together for five minutes before reducing it to a simmer. Cook for twenty minutes.

Heat a grill pan that's been greased over medium heat, and then add in your peaches to grill for one minute per side.

Heat the remaining ¾ cup of milk in your microwave. Cook the quinoa with a splash of milk, berries and grilled peaches. Don't forget to drizzle with honey before serving it.

Nutrition: Calories: 435

 Protein: 9.2

Grams Fat: 13.7

Grams Carbs: 24.9

Grams Sodium: 141 mg

Cholesterol: 78 mg

7. Eggs Benedict

Preparation Time: 15 minutes

Cooking Time: 15 minutes

Servings: 2

Ingredients:

One-half cup water

Two tomato slices

Three tbsp. sour cream, fat-free

One whole wheat English muffin, low-sodium

Two tsp. milk, fat-free

One tsp. mustard, low-sodium (See Helpful Tip below)

Two large eggs

One tbsp. chives, chopped

Two oz. ham slices, low-sodium

Olive oil cooking spray

Directions:

Adjust the stove temperature to broil. Prepare a flat sheet with a section of tin foil to use later.

Blend the sour cream, mustard, and milk in a glass dish and set to the side.

Slice the English muffin into two and set on the prepped flat sheet.

Heat in the stove for about two minutes.

In the meantime, use olive oil to coat a pan and then pour in the water.

Heat until it bubbles and then turn the burner down to low.

Open one of the eggs and put into an additional glass dish.

Slowly distribute the full egg to the simmering water, trying not to break the yolk.

Repeat steps 7 and 8 for the other egg and make sure they are not touching.

Warm for about 4 minutes.

Withdraw the muffins from the stove and layer the ham and tomato evenly on each of the muffins and broil for another 60 seconds.

Transfer the eggs with a spoon with holes and transfer to the prepared muffins.

Distribute the topping over the eggs liberally and dust with the chopped chives.

Serve immediately and enjoy!

Nutrition: Sodium: 502 mg Protein: 15 gm Fat: 8 gm Sugar: 5 gm Calories: 201

8. Fruit Smoothie

Preparation Time: 5 minutes

Cooking Time: 5 minutes

Servings: 1

Ingredients:

One-fourth cup blueberries

Four oz. strawberries

One-half orange, peeled

Four oz. papaya peeled, seeded and diced

One-fourth cup ice cubes

Four oz. soy milk

Directions:

Pulse the blueberries, strawberries, peeled orange, and milk in a blender for approximately half a minute.

Combine the ice cubes and papaya and continue to blend for another 30 seconds.

Transfer to a glass and enjoy immediately.

You can also use frozen fruit if you prefer.

Nutrition:

Sodium: 71e mg

Protein: 6 gm

Fat: 3 gm

Sugar: 26 gm

Calories: 184

9. Green Smoothie

Preparation Time: 5 minutes

Cooking Time: 5 minutes

Servings: 1

Ingredients:

One-fourth cup yogurt, non-fat and plain

One-half tsp. vanilla extract

One cup spinach

One medium banana

One-half cup milk, fat-free

Three-fourths cup mango

One-fourth cup whole oats

Directions:

Using a blender, combine the baby spinach, yogurt, whole oats, milk, and mango. Pulse for approximately half a minute.

Blend the banana and vanilla extract and pulse for an additional half minute until smooth.

Empty into a serving glass and enjoy immediately.

Nutrition:

Sodium: 20 mg

Protein: 2 gm

Fat: 0 gm

Sugar: 5 gm

Calories: 48

10.   Homemade Bacon

Preparation Time: 80 minutes

Cooking Time: 80 minutes

Servings: 4

Ingredients: One tsp. cumin seasoning - One tsp. black pepper - Two tbsp. olive oil

Sixteen oz. pork belly, sliced no more than one-fourth inch thick

Four tsp. liquid smoke - Two tsp. smoked paprika seasoning - Three tbsp. maple syrup

One-fourth tsp. salt

Directions:

Set your stove to the temperature of 200° Fahrenheit. Cover a flat sheet with a rim with foil. Set to the side.

Remove the rind from the pork belly slices by using kitchen scissors and arrange the slices on the prepped baking pan so they are in a single layer and not touching.

Utilize another pan if necessary depending on the thickness of your bacon.

In a glass dish, blend the maple syrup and the liquid smoke until integrated.

In a separate dish, combine the pepper, cumin, and smoked paprika fully.

Use a pastry brush to apply the maple syrup to each of the bacon slices.

Turn the slices over and repeat step 5.

Dust all of the slices with the mixed seasonings and rub the spices into the meat.

Heat in the stove for 60 minutes and remove.

The bacon is ready to be stored or fried. See the Helpful Tips below for storing instructions.

Empty the olive oil into a skillet and arrange the slices in a single layer. You will need to cook in stages.

Brown for approximately two minutes while turning over as needed to fully fry to your desired crispiness.

Remove to a paper towel covered plate and enjoy while hot!

Helpful Tips:

If you have thicker cut pork belly slices, you will only need one pan for this recipe. If you have the thinner cut slices, you will need to use two. They can be placed in the oven at the same time.

To store the pre-cooked bacon, set in a lidded tub for 5 days in the fridge.

If freezing, wrap in freezer or wax paper in between the slices and store for three months. Allow to defrost in the fridge at least 6 hours before frying.

Nutrition: Sodium: 122 mg Protein: 4 gm Fat: 24 gm Sugar: 4 gm Calories: 253

11.   Oatmeal Pancakes

Preparation Time: 30 minutes

Cooking Time: 30 minutes

Servings: 2

Ingredients: One-half tsp. ground cinnamon

4 oz. whole wheat flour - Two oz. oats, old fashioned

One tsp. baking powder, salt-free

One/eight tsp. salt

Olive oil cooking spray

4 oz. milk, skim

One/eight cup Greek yogurt, no-fat

One large egg

One-half tsp. vanilla extract

Three tsp. brown sugar

Directions:

In a big dish, blend the salt, whole wheat flour, ground cinnamon, whole oats, and baking powder combining completely.

Using another dish, fully integrate the milk and egg until the mixed well.

Combine the vanilla extract, yogurt, and brown sugar into the eggs and whisk to remove any lumpiness.

Slowly empty the egg dish into the flour dish making sure it is totally combined but do not mix too thoroughly.

Warm a skillet. Make sure the skillet is sprayed with olive oil.

Distribute approximately a quarter of the batter into the skillet.

Turn the pancake over after the top starts to bubble after about 60 seconds.

Let the pancake cook for approximately another minute and flip as needed until browned completely.

Remove to a plate and coat the skillet with an additional coat of olive oil spray.

Perform steps 6 through 9 until all the pancakes are finished.

Serve while hot and enjoy!

Helpful Tip:

If you would like to be creative with this recipe, combine one-fourth cup of fruit into the batter before transferring to the hot skillet. Of course, you can add your fruits on top before serving.

Nutrition: Sodium: 116 mg Protein: 9 gm Fat: 3 gm Sugar: 6 gm Calories: 150

Chapter 11   Snack and Appetizers Recipes

12.   Homemade Spinach Artichoke Dip

Preparation Time: 15 minutes

Cooking Time: 10 minutes

Servings: 16

Ingredients: 1 1/4 cups raw cashews - 1 tsp olive oil - 5 cloves garlic, peeled

3/4 cup chopped shallot - 1 1/2 cups unsweetened almond milk

5 tbsp nutritional yeast, for cheesy flavor - 1/2 tsp black pepper

1 tsp coconut aminos

2 tbsp water

4 cups loosely packed chopped fresh spinach

1 14-ounce can artichoke hearts, rinsed, drained well, and roughly chopped

2 tbsp fat free parmesan cheese

4 large whole wheat pita bread, quartered

Directions:

Place cashews in a bowl, cover with boiling water and let it soak for an hour. Then drain well.

Place a cast iron pan on medium fire and heat oil. Add garlic and cook for a minute. Stir in shallots and cook for 4 minutes or until soft.

In a blender, add half of garlic and shallot mixture. Add drained cashews, almond milk, nutritional yeast, pepper, and coconut aminos. Puree until smooth and creamy. Scrape sides of blender and blend once more.

Preheat oven to 350oF.

Return same cast iron pan to medium fire and add water, spinach, and artichoke hearts. Cook until spinach is wilted, around 4 minutes.

Pour pureed mixture into pan and mix well. Turn off fire. Sprinkle cheese on top.

Pop in the oven and bake for 8 minutes.

Serve with your favorite bread or cracker.

Nutrition:

Calories: 108 Protein: 5.2g Carbs: 15.6g Fat: 3.5g Saturated Fat: 0.6g

Sodium: 209 mg

13. Pumpkin Walnut Cookie

Preparation Time: 35 minutes

Cooking Time: 30 minutes

Servings: 24

Ingredients:

1 tbsp baking powder

½ tsp salt

1½ tsp pumpkin pie spice mix

1¼ cups whole wheat flour

1½ cups flour

½ cup vegetable oil

2 eggs

1 cup brown sugar

3 packets Stevia

1 ¾ cups pumpkin, cooked and pureed (15 oz. can)

1 cup walnuts or hazelnuts, chopped

1 cup raisin

Directions:

Grease a cookie sheet with cooking spray and preheat oven to 400oF.

In a medium bowl mix baking powder, salt, pumpkin pie spice mix, whole wheat flour, and flour.

In a large bowl beat eggs and oil thoroughly.

Add in brown sugar and stevia beat for at least 3 minutes.

Mix in pumpkin puree and beat well.

Slowly add the dry ingredients beating well after each addition.

Fold in nuts and raisins.

Using a 1 tbsp measuring spoon, get two salt spoonfuls of the dough and place on cookie sheet at least an inch apart. With the bottom of a spoon, flatten cookie.

Pop into the oven and bake until golden brown, around 10 minutes.

Once done, remove from oven, serve and enjoy or store in tightly lidded containers for up to a week.

Nutrition: Calories: 230.4 Protein: 5.8g Carbs: 22.1g Fat: 13.2g Saturated Fat: 5g Sodium: 82mg

14.   Choco-Chip Cookies with Walnuts and Oatmeal

Preparation Time: 20 minutes

Cooking Time: 16 minutes

Servings: 24

Ingredients: ½ tsp salt - ½ tsp baking soda - 1 tsp ground cinnamon

½ cup whole wheat pastry flour - ½ cup all-purpose flour

2 cups rolled oats (not quick cooking) - 4 tbsp cold unsalted butter, cut into pieces

½ cup tahini - 2/3 cup packed light brown sugar - 6 packets Stevia - 1 tbsp vanilla extract

1 large egg white - 1 large egg

½ cup chopped walnuts

1 cup semisweet Choco chips

Directions:

Position two racks in the middle of the oven, leaving at least a 3-inch space in between them. Preheat oven to 350oF and grease baking sheets with cooking spray.

In medium bowl, whisk together salt, baking soda, cinnamon, whole wheat flour, all-purpose flour and oats.

In a large bowl, with a mixer beat butter and tahini until well combined.

Add brown sugar and Stevia, mixing continuously until creamy.

Mix in vanilla, egg white and egg and beat for a minute.

Cup by cup mix in the dry ingredients until well incorporated.

Fold in walnuts and Choco chips.

Get two tablespoonfuls of the batter and roll with your moistened hands into a ball.

Evenly place balls into prepped baking sheets at least an inch apart.

Pop in the oven and bake for 16 minutes. Ten minutes into baking time, switch pans from top to bottom and bottom to top. Continue baking for 6 more minutes.

Remove from oven, cool on a wire rack. Allow pans to cool completely before adding the next batch of cookies to be baked.

Cookies can be stored for up to 10 days in a tightly sealed container or longer in the fridge.

Nutrition:

Calories: 150.6 Protein: 3.8g Carbs: 15.4g Fat: 8.2g Saturated Fat: 2.8g Sodium: 87mg

15.   Potato Casserole

Preparation Time: 25 minutes

Cook Time: 20 minutes

Servings: 10

Ingredients:

1 tsp dried dill weed

¼ tsp black pepper

¼ cup green onions, chopped

2 tbsp olive oil

16 small new potatoes, around 5 cups

Directions:

Using water and vegetable brush clean all potatoes.

For about 20 minutes, boil potatoes then drain and cool them for 20 minutes.

Mix spices, onions, and olive oil. Then cut potatoes into quarters and combine with the mixture.

Refrigerate and enjoy!

Nutrition:

Calories: 237

Protein: 5.6g

Carbs: 46.9g

Fat: 3.0g

Saturated Fat: .4g

Sodium: 22.5mg

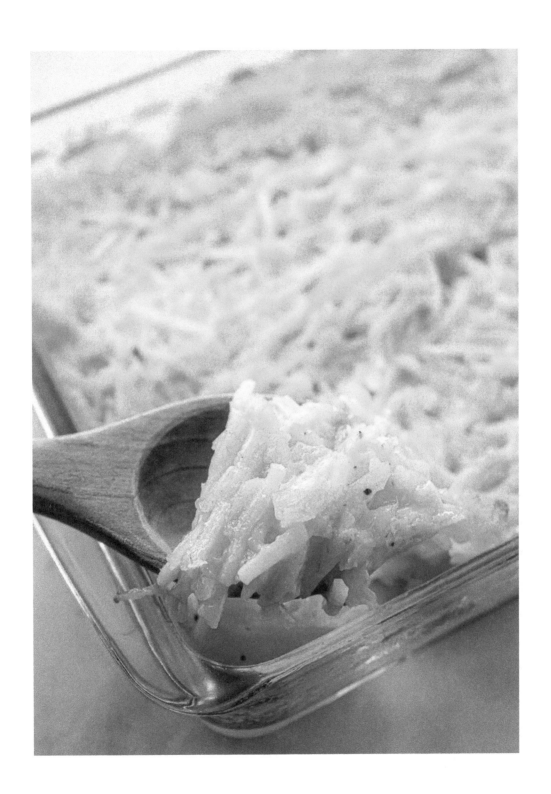

16.   Cornbread with Southern Twist

Preparation Time: 25 minutes

Cooking Time: 20 minutes

Servings: 8

Ingredients:

1 tbsp olive oil

1 ¼ cups skim milk

¼ cup egg substitute

4 tbsp sodium free baking powder

½ cup flour

1 ½ cups cornmeal

Directions:

Prepare 8 x 8-inch baking dish or a black iron skillet then add shortening.

Put the baking dish or skillet inside the oven on 425oF and leave there for 10 minutes.

In a bowl, add milk and egg then mix well.

Take out the skillet and add the heated oil into the batter and stir well.

Once all ingredients are mixed, pour mixture into skillet.

Then cook for 15 to 20 minutes in the oven until golden brown.

Nutrition:

Calories: 206.7

Protein: 4.9g

Carbs: 38g

Fat: 3.9g

Saturated Fat: .9g

Sodium: 40mg

17.   Deviled Eggs Guac Style

Preparation Time: 10 minutes

Cook Time: 0 minutes

Servings: 12

Ingredients:

1 ripe avocado

1 tbsp green onion, chopped

1 tbsp Cilantro

1 tbsp Lime

1/2 jalapeno chili pepper

1 tbsp light sour cream

6 medium eggs, hard boiled and peeled

Directions:

In a medium bowl, mash avocado. Mix in green onion, cilantro, lime, pepper, and sour cream. Mix well.

Slice hard boiled eggs in half lengthwise.

Scoop out yolk and place in bowl of avocados. Mix well.

Scoop out avocado yolk mixture and spoon into egg white holes.

Serve and enjoy or refrigerate for future use.

Nutrition:

Calories: 60

Protein: 3.1g

Carbs: 1.8g

Fat: 4.7g

Saturated Fat: 1.1g

Sodium: 34mg

18.   Buffalo Chicken Dip

Preparation Time: 15 minutes

Cooking Time: 10 minutes

Servings: 8

Ingredients:

1-piece chicken breast half, sliced into strips

½ cup cottage cheese, fat free

1 tbsp ranch dressing

2 tbsp hot sauce

¼ cup low fat cheddar cheese

6 stalks celery, cut into 4-inch lengths

Directions:

Place a fry pan on medium fire and pan fry chicken pieces until cooked, around 8 minutes.

Stir in ranch dressing, hot sauce, and cheddar cheese until melted.

Turn off fire and transfer to a bowl. Mix in cottage cheese and stir well.

Serve with celery sticks on the side.

Nutrition:

Calories: 71

Protein: 8.7g

Carbs: 1.3g

Fat: 3.3g

Saturated Fat: 1.3g

Sodium: 290 mg

19.   Ricotta and Pomegranate Bruschetta

Preparation Time: 15 minutes

Cooking Time: 12 minutes

Servings: 12

Ingredients:

6 slice Whole Grain Nut Bread

1 cup Low Fat Ricotta Cheese

1/2 tsp Grated lemon zest

1/2 cup Pomegranate Arils

2 tsp Thyme, Fresh

Directions:

Toast bread until lightly browned.

Meanwhile, in a small bowl whisk well cheese and lemon zest.

Slice the toasted bread in half. Slather top with cottage cheese.

Top with thyme and pomegranate.

Serve and enjoy.

Nutrition:

Calories: 69

Protein: 4.1g

Carbs: 11.1g

Fat: 1.0g S

aturated Fat: 0.2g

Sodium: 123mg

20.   Crab Stuffed Mushrooms

Preparation Time: 30 minutes

Cooking Time: 25 minutes

Servings: 6

Ingredients: 2 tbsp minced green onion - 1 cup cooked crabmeat, chopped finely

¼ cup Monterey Jack cheese, shredded, low fat - 1 tsp lemon juice

½ tsp dill - 1 lb. fresh button mushrooms

Directions:

De stem mushrooms, wash and drain well.

Chop mushroom stems.

Preheat oven to 400oF and lightly grease a baking pan with cooking spray.

In a small bowl, whisk well green onion, crabmeat, lemon juice, dill, and chopped mushroom stems.

Evenly spread mushrooms on prepared pan with cap sides up. Evenly spoon crab meat mixture on top of mushroom caps.

Pop in the oven and bake for 20 minutes.

Remove from oven and sprinkle cheese on top.

Return to oven and broil for 3 minutes.

Serve and enjoy.

Nutrition:

Calories: 58

Protein: 8.2g

Carbs: 3.8g

Fat: 1.6g

Saturated Fat: 0.8g

Sodium: 128mg

21. Sour Cream and Onion Dip Carrot Sticks

Preparation Time: 5 minutes

Cooking Time: 0 minutes

Servings: 8

Ingredients:

1 sweet onion, peeled and minced

½ cup sour cream

2 tbsp low fat mayonnaise

4 stalks celery, cut into 3-inch lengths

2 cups carrot sticks

Directions:

In a bowl, whisk well sour cream and mayonnaise until thoroughly combined.

Stir in onion and mix well.

Let it sit for an hour in the fridge and serve with carrot and celery sticks on the side.

Nutrition:

Calories: 60

Protein: 1.6g

Carbs: 7.2g

Fat: 3.1g

Saturated Fat: 1.7g

Sodium: 38 mg

Chapter 12 Lunch Recipes

22.   Cheesy Black Bean Wraps

Preparation Time: 15 Minutes

Cooking Time: 15 Minutes

Servings: 6

Ingredients: 2 Tablespoons Green Chili Peppers, Chopped

4 Green Onions, Diced - 1 Tomato, Diced - 1 Tablespoon Garlic, Chopped

6 Tortilla Wraps, Whole Grain & Fat Free - ¾ Cup Cheddar Cheese, Shredded

¾ Cup Salsa - 1 ½ Cups Corn Kernels - 3 Tablespoons Cilantro, Fresh & Chopped

1 ½ Cup Black Beans, Canned & Drained

Directions:

Toss your chili peppers, corn, black beans, garlic, tomato, onions and cilantro in a bowl.

Heat the mixture in a microwave for a minute, and stir for a half a minute. Spread the two tortillas between paper towels and microwave for twenty seconds. Warm the remaining tortillas the same way, and add a half a cup of bean mixture, two tablespoons of salsa and two tablespoons of cheese for each tortilla. Roll them up before serving.

Nutrition:

Calories: 341

Protein: 19

Grams Fat: 11

Grams Carbs: 36.5

Grams Sodium: 141 mg

Cholesterol: 0 mg

23.   Arugula Risotto

Preparation Time: 25 Minutes

Cooking Time: 25 Minutes

Servings: 4

Ingredients:1 Tablespoon Olive Oil - ½ Cup Yellow Onion, Chopped

1 Cup Quinoa, Rinsed - 1 Clove Garlic, Minced - 2 ½ Cups Vegetable Stock, Low Sodium

2 Cups Arugula, Chopped & Stemmed

1 Carrot, Peeled & shredded

½ Cup Shiitake Mushrooms, Sliced

¼ Teaspoon Black Pepper

¼ Teaspoon Sea Salt, Fine

¼ Cup Parmesan Cheese, Grated

Directions:

Get a saucepan and place it over medium heat, heating up your oil. Cook for four minutes until your onions are softened, and then add in your garlic and quinoa. Cook for a minute.

Stir in your stock, and bring it to a boil. Reduce it to simmer, and cook for twelve minutes.

Add in your arugula, mushrooms and carrots, cooking for an additional two minutes.

Add in salt, pepper and cheese before serving.

Nutrition:

Calories: 288

Protein: 6

Grams Fat: 5

Grams Carbs: 28

Grams Sodium: 739 mg

Cholesterol: 0.5 mg

24. Vegetarian Stuffed Eggplant

Preparation Time: 35 Minutes

Cooking Time: 35 Minutes

Servings: 2

Ingredients:

4 Ounces White Beans, Cooked

1 Tablespoons Olive Oil

1 cup Water

1 Eggplant

¼ Cup Onion, Chopped

½ Cup Bell Pepper, Chopped

1 Cup Canned Tomatoes, Unsalted

¼ Cup Tomato Liquid

¼ Cup Celery, Chopped

1 Cup Mushrooms, Fresh & Sliced

¾ Cup Breadcrumbs, Whole Wheat

Black Pepper to Taste

Directions:

Preheat the oven to 350, and then grease a baking dish with cooking spray.

Trim the eggplant and cut it in half lengthwise. Scoop the pulp out using a spoon, leaving a shell that's a quarter of an inch thick.

Place the shells in the baking dish with their cut side up.

Add the water to the bottom of the dish, and dice the eggplant pulp into cubes, setting them to the side.

Add the oil into an iron skillet, heating it over medium heat.

Stir in peppers, chopped eggplants, and onions with your celery, mushrooms, tomatoes and tomato juice.

Cook for ten minutes on simmering heat, and then stir in your bread crumbs, beans and black pepper. Divide the mixture between eggshells.

Cover with foil, and bake for fifteen minutes. Serve warm.

Nutrition:

Calories: 334 Protein: 26 Grams Fat: 10 Grams

Carbs: 35 Grams Sodium: 142 mg Cholesterol: 162 mg

25.   Vegetable Tacos

Preparation Time: 30 Minutes

Cooking Time: 30 Minutes

Servings: 4

Ingredients:

1 Tablespoon Olive Oil

1 Cup Red Onion, Chopped

1 Cup Yellow Summer Squash, Diced

1 Cup Green Zucchini, Diced

3 Cloves Garlic, Minced

4 Tomatoes, Seeded & Chopped

1 Jalapeno Chili, Seeded & Chopped

1 Cup Corn Kernels, Fresh

1 Cup Pinto Beans, Canned, Rinsed & Drained

½ Cup Cilantro, Fresh & Chopped

8 Corn Tortillas

½ Cup Smoke Flavored Salsa

Directions:

Get out a saucepan and add in your olive oil over medium heat, and stir in your onion. Cook until softened.

Add in your squash and zucchini, cooking for an additional five minutes.

Stir in your garlic, beans, tomatoes, jalapeño and corn. Cook for an additional five minutes before stirring in your cilantro and removing the pan from heat.

Warm each tortilla, in a nonstick skillet for twenty seconds per side.

Place the tortillas on a serving plate, spooning the vegetable mixture into each. Top with salsa, and roll to serve.

Nutrition:

Calories: 310

Protein: 10 Grams

Fat: 6 Grams

Carbs: 54 Grams Sodium: 97 mg

Cholesterol: 20 mg

26.   Tuscan Stew

Preparation Time: 1 Hour 40 Minutes

Cooking Time: 1 Hour 40 Minutes

Servings: 6

Ingredients:

Croutons:

1 Tablespoons Olive Oil - 1 Slice Bread, Whole Grain & Cubed - 2 Cloves Garlic, Quartered

Soup:

1 Bay Leaf - 2 Cups White Beans, Soaked Overnight & Drained - 6 Cups Water

½ Teaspoon Sea Salt, Divided - 1 Cup Yellow Onion, Chopped - 2 Tablespoons Olive Oil

3 Carrots, Peeled & Chopped - 6 Cloves Garlic, Chopped

¼ Teaspoon Ground Black Pepper - 1 Tablespoons Rosemary, Fresh & Chopped

1 ½ Cups Vegetable Stock

Directions:

Add your oil to a skillet and heat it, and then cook your garlic for a minute. It should become fragrant. Allow it to sit for ten minutes before removing your garlic from the oil.

Return the pan with the oil to heat and then throw in your bread cubes. Cook for five minutes. They should be golden, and then set them to the side.

Mix your salt, water, bay leaf and white beans in the pot, boiling on high heat before reducing to a simmer.

Cover the beans and cook for one hour to one hour and ten minutes. They should be al dente.

Drain the beans, but reserve a half a cup of the cooking liquid. Discard the bay leaf, and transfer your beans to a bowl.

Mix the reserved liquid with ½ cup of beans, returning it to a boil. Mash with a fork to form a paste, and then place the pot on the stove. Heat the oil using the pot.

Add in your onions and carrots. Cook for seven minutes and add garlic, and then cook for a minute more. Add in your rosemary, salt, pepper, stock and bean mixture.

Allow it to come to a boil and then reduce the heat to let it simmer. Let it simmer for five minutes, and then top with croutons. Garnish with rosemary sprigs and enjoy.

Nutrition:

Calories: 307 Protein: 16 Grams Fat: 7 Grams Carbs: 45 Grams Sodium: 463 mg Cholesterol: 68 mg

27.   Simple Pasta Limon

Preparation Time: 15 Minutes

Cooking Time: 15 minutes

Servings: 2

Ingredients:

1/2-pound angel hair whole wheat spaghetti, cooked

1 lemon, juiced and zested

3 1/2 ounces low-sodium parmesan cheese

Freshly ground black pepper

1 tablespoon olive oil

¼ cup packed fresh basil leaves, torn

Directions:

Cook angel hair pasta according to manufacturer's instructions minus the oil and salt.

Meanwhile in a large bowl, mix well all remaining ingredients.

Once pasta is cooked, reserve ¼ cup of the boiling liquid, and drain pasta well.

Add pasta to bowl of cheese and swirl to coat. If needed, add a tbsp of the reserved boiling water to un-thicken sauce.

Serve and enjoy.

Nutrition:

Calories: 429

Protein: 26.8g

Carbs: 33.6g

Fat: 22.3g

Saturated Fat: 10.5g

Sodium: 35mg

28.   Baked Salmon with Dill 'n Garlic

Preparation Time: 15 minutes

Cooking Time: 15 minutes

Servings: 4

Ingredients:

2 8-oz. salmon filets, skin on

1 tbsp avocado oil

1 pinch black pepper

4 tbsp fresh dill, chopped, divided

1 small lemon, thinly sliced into 1/8th-inch rounds

1/4 cup hummus

2 tbsp lemon juice

2 cloves garlic, minced

Directions:

Lightly grease a non-stick baking dish with cooking spray and preheat oven to 400oF.

Place fish on baking sheet and drizzle with oil. Season with pepper and 2 tbsp fresh dill. Top fish with thinly sliced lemon.

Pop in the oven and roast for 15 minutes or until flaky.

Meanwhile, make the dill-garlic sauce by pulsing in a blender the garlic, remaining dill, and lemon juice until creamy. Stir in hummus.

Serve salmon topped with dill-garlic sauce.

Nutrition:

Calories: 486.4

Protein: 70.7g

Carbs: 8.6g

Fat: 18.8g

Saturated Fat: 3.6g

Sodium: 97mg

29.   Pan-Fried Kale Falafel

Preparation Time: 15 minutes

Cooking Time: 15 minutes

Servings: 4

Ingredients: 4 large cloves garlic, peeled - 3 tbsp fresh lemon juice - 1 tsp coconut aminos

4 cups loosely packed kale, stems removed and torn

1 15-ounce can chickpeas, rinsed well and drained

1 ½ tbsp tahini - 1/2 tsp ground cumin - 1/3 cup oat flour - 1 tbsp olive oil

Directions:

In a blender, add garlic, lemon juice, and coconut aminos. Puree until smooth and creamy or garlic are chopped finely.

Add kale and blend until finely chopped, but not creamy.

Add chickpeas, tahini and cumin. Blend well until chickpeas finely crumbled.

With a spatula, scrape the side of blender. And blend one last time.

Transfer to a bowl. Fold in oat flour.

Evenly divide batter into 4. Form into a ¼ to ½-inch thick patty.

On medium low fire, place a large nonstick pan and heat oil. Swirl oil to coat pan. After 2 minutes of heating add the patties and cook for 3 to 4 minutes per side or until golden brown. Flip and cook the other side.

Serve and enjoy.

Nutrition: Calories: 296.2

Protein: 11.9g

Carbs: 38.3g

Fat: 10.6g

Saturated Fat: 1.3g

Sodium: 319mg

30. Stir-Fried Brussels Sprouts Korean Style

Preparation Time: 15 minutes

Cooking Time: 15 minutes

Servings: 8

Ingredients:

1/2 cup Korean Gochujang Sauce

1 tsp sesame oil

2 tsp coconut aminos, divided

1 tbsp maple syrup

2 - 3 tbsp water

7 heaped cups halved Brussels sprouts

1 stalk green onion, chopped

Directions:

In a small bowl, whisk well gochujang sauce, sesame oil, 1 tsp coconut aminos, and maple syrup. Mix well and set aside.

Place a large nonstick saucepan on medium high fire.

Add Brussels sprouts and water. Cover and cook for 5 minutes.

Stir fry Brussels sprouts until water is fully evaporated.

Mix in sauce and stir fry until heated through and Brussels sprouts are crisp tender. If needed, add another tbsp of water to continue cooking.

Serve and enjoy.

Nutrition:

Calories: 58

Protein: 2.9g

Carbs: 9.8g

Fat: .8g

Saturated Fat: 1g

Sodium: 136mg

31.   Tuna-Pasta Salad

Preparation Time: 15 minutes

Cooking Time: 15 minutes

Servings: 4

Ingredients: 2 cups whole wheat macaroni, uncooked

2 5-oz cans low-sodium tuna, water pack - 1/3 cup diced onion

¼ cup sliced carrots

½ cup chopped zucchini

¼ cup fat free mayonnaise

¼ cup light sour cream

¼ tsp pepper

Directions:

In a pot of boiling water, cook macaroni according to manufacturer's instructions minus the oil and salt.

Drain macaroni, run under cold tap water until cool and set aside.

Drain tuna and discard liquid.

Place tuna in a salad bowl.

Add zucchini, carrots, drained macaroni and onion. Toss to mix.

Add mayonnaise and sour cream. Mix well.

Season with pepper, serve and enjoy.

Serve and enjoy.

Nutrition:

Calories: 174.4

Protein: 5.1g

Carbs: 27.7g

Fat: 4.8g S

aturated Fat: 1.5g

Sodium: 54mg

Chapter 13   Dinner Recipes

32.   Red Lentil and Cauliflower Curry

Preparation Time: 40 minutes

Cooking Time: 40 minutes

Servings: 4

Ingredients: 1 ½ cups water - 2/3 cup red lentils - 1 tsp whole mustard seed - 1 tsp whole cumin seed

1 tsp whole coriander seed - 3 whole cardamom pods - 1 tsp avocado oil

1/2 cup sliced shallot - 1 ½ tbsp minced ginger - 1 serrano pepper, seeds removed and diced

2 cloves garlic, minced - 3 large ripe tomatoes, chopped

1 ½ cups peeled and chopped golden potato or sweet potato, ½-inch cubes

1 cup chopped cauliflower - 1 cup chopped red bell pepper - 1 tsp curry powder

1 ½ cups low sodium vegetable broth - 2 tbsp coconut aminos - 1 packet stevia - 1/2 cup almond milk

Directions:

In a small pot, bring water to a boil and add lentil. Cook uncovered until just tender, around 9 minutes. Drain and set aside.

Place a large nonstick pot on medium flame and toast mustard, cumin, coriander, and cardamom pods for 2 to 3 minutes or until fragrant and popping.

In same pot, add oil and swirl to coat pot. Stir in shallot, ginger, pepper, and garlic. Sauté for 5 minutes until shallots are soft and translucent.

Stir in chopped tomatoes. Cook for 5 minutes.

Add sweet potatoes and continue sautéing for 7 minutes until tomatoes are pureed looking. If needed add a tablespoon of water to deglaze pot.

Stir in cauliflower, bell pepper, curry powder, coconut aminos, drained lentil, and stevia. Mix well and cook for 5 minutes.

Add vegetable broth and bring to a simmer. Continue cooking for 5 minutes or until veggies are tender.

Turn off fire and stir in almond milk.

Serve and enjoy.

Nutrition:

Calories: 234.6 Protein: 11.8g Carbs: 39.2g Fat: 3.4g

Saturated Fat: .5g Sodium: 105mg

33.   Black Bean Soup

Preparation Time: 25 minutes

Cooking Time: 25 minutes

Servings: 4

Ingredients: 1 tsp olive oil

3 cloves garlic, minced

1 cup diced white or yellow onion

2 tsp ground cumin

1 ½ tsp chili powder

1/4 tsp ground coriander

1-2 chipotle peppers in adobo sauce, drained well

2 15-ounce cans black beans, rinsed and drained well

2 cups low sodium vegetable broth

3 tbsp chopped dark chocolate

2 tbsp chopped cilantro

1 lime cut into wedges

Directions:

Place large nonstick pot on medium fire and heat oil. Swirl oil to coat pan and add garlic. Cook for a minute.

Stir in onion and cook for 3 minutes.

Stir in cumin, chili powder, and coriander. Continue sautéing for a minute or two.

Add chipotle peppers and black beans. Sauté for 3 minutes or until heated through.

Stir in chocolate and cook for 2 minutes until starting to melt.

Stir in broth. Mix well and bring to a simmer. Once simmering, lower fire and simmer for 5 minutes.

Transfer to bowls, garnish with cilantro and lime wedges.

Serve and enjoy.

Nutrition:

Calories: 353.5

Protein: 20.8g

Carbs: 60.6g

Fat: 3.1g

Saturated Fat: .6g Sodium: 105mg

34. Avocado-Orange Grilled Chicken

Preparation Time: 15 minutes

Cooking Time: 15 minutes

Servings: 4

Ingredients:

1 tbsp honey

2 tbsp chopped cilantro

¼ cup minced red onion

1 cup low fat yogurt

1-lb boneless, skinless chicken breasts

½ tsp pepper

¼ tsp salt

¼ cup fresh lime juice

1 avocado

1 small red onion, sliced thinly

2 oranges, peeled and sectioned

Directions:

In a large bowl mix honey, cilantro, minced red onion and yogurt.

Marinate chicken in mixture for at least 30 minutes.

Grease grate and preheat grill to medium high fire.

Remove chicken from marinade and season with pepper and salt.

Grill for 6 minutes per side or until chicken is cooked and juices run clear.

Meanwhile, peel avocado and discard seed. Chop avocados and place in bowl. Quickly add lime juice and toss avocado to coat well with juice.

Add cilantro, thinly sliced onions and oranges into bowl of avocado, mix well.

Serve grilled chicken and avocado dressing on the side.

Nutrition:

Calories: 356.8 Protein: 15.2g Carbs: 40.7g
Fat: 14.8g Saturated Fat: 3.5g Sodium: 497mg

35. American Cheese over Herbed Portobello Mushrooms

Preparation Time: 10 minutes

Cooking Time: 10 minutes

Servings: 2

Ingredients:

2 Portobello mushrooms, stemmed and wiped clean

1 tsp minced garlic

¼ tsp dried rosemary

1 tbsp brown sugar

½ cup balsamic vinegar

¼ cup grated non-fat American cheese

Directions:

In oven, position rack 4-inches away from the top and preheat broiler.

Prepare a baking dish by spraying with cooking spray lightly.

Stemless, place mushroom gill side up.

Mix well garlic, rosemary, brown sugar and vinegar in a small bowl.

Drizzle over mushrooms equally.

Marinate for at least 5 minutes before popping into the oven and broiling for 4 minutes per side or until tender.

Once cooked, remove from oven, sprinkle cheese, return to broiler and broil for a minute or two or until cheese melts.

Remove from oven and serve right away.

Nutrition:

Calories: 131.2

Protein: 8.7g

Carbs: 19.6g

Fat: 2g

Saturated Fat: .9g
Sodium: 342mg

36.   Garden Salad with Oranges 'n Olives

Preparation Time: 15 minutes

Cooking Time: 15 minutes

Servings: 4

Ingredients:

1 tbsp finely chopped celery

1 tbsp finely chopped red onion

1 tbsp extra virgin olive oil

4 garlic cloves, minced

½ cup red wine vinegar

4 boneless, skinless chicken breasts, 4-oz each

2 garlic cloves

8 cups leaf lettuce, washed and dried

2 navel oranges, peeled and segmented

16 large ripe black olives

¼ tsp freshly cracked black pepper or more to taste

Directions:

Prepare the dressing by mixing pepper, celery, onion, olive oil, garlic and vinegar in a small bowl. Whisk well to combine.

Lightly grease grate and preheat grill to high.

Rub chicken with the garlic cloves and discard garlic.

Grill chicken for 5 minutes per side or until cooked through.

Remove from grill and let it stand for 5 minutes before cutting into ½-inch strips.

In 4 serving plates, evenly arrange two cups lettuce, ¼ of the sliced oranges and 4 olives per plate.

Top each plate with ¼ serving of grilled chicken, evenly drizzle with dressing, and topped with pepper.

Serve and enjoy.

Nutrition:

Calories: 96.3 Protein: 3.3g Carbs: 9.3g

Fat: 5.1g Saturated Fat: 1g Sodium: 241mg

37. Roasted Vegetables with Polenta

Preparation Time: 35 minutes

Cooking Time: 35 minutes

Servings: 6

Ingredients: 1 sweet red pepper, seeded, cored and cut into chunks - 6 medium mushrooms, sliced

1 small green zucchini, cut into ¼-inch slices - 1 small yellow zucchini, cut into ¼-inch slices

1 small eggplant, peeled and cut into ¼-inch slices - 10-oz frozen spinach, thawed

1 ½ cups coarse polenta - 6 cups water - ¼ tsp cracked black pepper

1 tbsp + 1 tsp extra virgin olive oil, divided - 10 ripe olives, chopped

6 dry-packed sun-dried tomatoes, soaked in water to rehydrate, drained and chopped

2 Roma tomatoes, sliced - 2 tsp oregano

Directions:

Grease a baking sheet and a 12-inch round baking dish, position oven rack 4-inches away from heat source and preheat broiler.

Place red pepper, mushrooms, zucchini and eggplant in prepared baking sheet in a single layer. Pop in the broiler and broil under low setting.

Turn the veggies after 5 minutes. Continue broiling until veggies are slightly browned and tender, another 3 minutes.

Wash and drain spinach. Set aside.

Preheat oven to 350oF.

Bring water to a boil in a medium saucepan.

Whisk in polenta and lower fire to a simmer. For 5 minutes, cook and stir.

Once polenta no longer sticks to pan, add 1/8 tsp pepper and 1 tbsp olive oil. Mix well and turn off fire.

Evenly spread polenta on base of prepped baking dish. Brush tops with 1 tsp olive oil and for ten minutes bake in the oven.

When done, remove polenta from oven and keep warm.

With paper towels remove excess water from spinach. Layer spinach on top of polenta followed by sliced tomatoes, olives, sun-dried tomatoes, and roasted veggies. Season with remaining pepper and oregano.

Bake for another 10 minutes.

Remove from oven, cut into equal servings and enjoy.

Nutrition: Calories: 72.7 Protein: 3.9g Carbs: 11.8g Fat: 1.1g Saturated Fat: .2g Sodium: 114mg

38.   Herbed and Spiced Grilled Eggplant

Preparation Time: 20 minutes

Cooking Time: 20 minutes

Servings: 4

Ingredients: 1 large aubergine eggplant, around 1 ½ lbs. - Pinch of ground cloves

Pinch of ground nutmeg - Pinch of ground ginger

½ tsp curry powder - ½ tsp ground coriander - ½ tsp ground cumin - 1 tsp mustard seed

1 tbsp olive oil

½ yellow onion, finely chopped

1 tbsp chopped fresh cilantro

1 tsp red wine vinegar

1 garlic clove, minced

1 tbsp light molasses

2 cups cherry tomatoes, halved

¼ tsp freshly ground black pepper

1 tsp coconut aminos

Directions:

Grease grill grate with cooking spray and preheat grill to high heat.

Trim eggplant and slice in ¼-inch thick lengthwise strips.

Grill strips of eggplant for 5 minutes per side or until browned and tender.

Remove eggplants from fire and keep warm.

In a small bowl, mix cloves, nutmeg, ginger, curry, coriander, cumin and mustard seed.

On medium high fire, place a medium nonstick skillet and heat oil.

Sauté spice mixture for 30 seconds and add onions.

Sauté onions for 4 minutes or until soft and translucent.

Add vinegar, garlic, molasses and tomatoes. Sauté for 4 minutes or until thickened.

Season with pepper and coconut aminos. Turn off fire.

On four plates, evenly divide grilled eggplant.

Evenly top each plate of eggplant with herbed and spiced sauce.

Serve and enjoy while warm.

Nutrition: Calories: 102.3 Protein: 1.5g Carbs: 12.6g Fat: 5.1g Saturated Fat: .7g Sodium: 8mg

39.   Low Sodium Shepherd's Pie

Preparation Time: 50 minutes

Cooking Time: 50 minutes

Servings: 6

Ingredients:

2 large baking potatoes, peeled and diced

½ cup skim milk

1 clove garlic, minced

1 medium onion, chopped

1 lb. lean ground beef

1 tsp coconut aminos

2 tbsp flour

¾ cup reduced sodium beef broth

4 cups frozen mixed vegetables

Pepper to taste

½ cup shredded fat free American cheese

Directions:

In a saucepan, bring to boil potatoes with water barely covering it.

Once boiling, reduce fire to a simmer and cook for 10 minutes or until soft while covered.

Once soft, drain potatoes, transfer to a bowl and mash. Add milk and mix well.

Preheat oven to 375oF.

In a large skillet, grease with cooking spray and sauté garlic and onions for a minute. Add ground meat and coconut aminos. Sauté until browned around 8 to 10 minutes.

Add flour and sauté for another minute.

Add broth and mixed vegetables. Season well with pepper. Sauté until bubbly, around 5 minutes.

Transfer mixture into an 8-inch square baking dish. Cover the top with mashed potato mixture and sprinkle cheese on top.

Pop into the oven and bake until bubbly around 25 minutes.

Serve and enjoy.

Nutrition: Calories: 439.4 Protein: 33g Carbs: 44.9g Fat: 14.2g Saturated Fat: 5.6g Sodium: 398mg

40.   Dijon Mustard and Lime Marinated Shrimp

Preparation Time: 10 minutes

Cooking Time: 10 minutes

Servings: 4

Ingredients:

½ tsp hot sauce

1 tbsp capers

1 tbsp Dijon mustard

½ cup fresh lime juice, plus lime zest as garnish

1 medium red onion, chopped

1 bay leaf

3 whole cloves

½ cup rice vinegar

1 cup water

1 lb. uncooked shrimp, peeled and deveined

Directions:

Mix hot sauce, mustard, capers, lime juice and onion in a shallow baking dish and set aside.

Bring to a boil in a large saucepan bay leaf, cloves, vinegar and water.

Once boiling, add shrimps and cook for a minute while stirring continuously.

Drain shrimps and pour shrimps into onion mixture.

For an hour, refrigerate while covered.

Then serve shrimps cold and garnished with lime zest.

Nutrition:

Calories: 118

Protein: 23.3g

Carbs: 3.7g

Fat: 1.7g

Saturated Fat: 0.1g
Sodium: 248mg

41.   Fennel Sauce Tenderloin

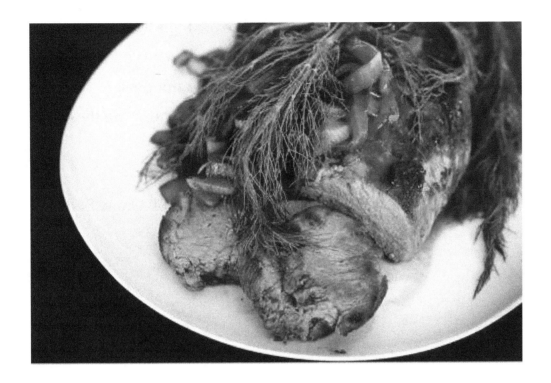

Preparation Time: 35 Minutes

Cooking Time: 35 Minutes

Servings: 4

Ingredients: 1 Fennel Bulb, Cored & Sliced - 1 Sweet Onion, Sliced

½ Cup Dry White Wine - 1 Teaspoon Fennel Seeds - 4 Pork Tenderloin Fillets

2 Tablespoons Olive Oil - 12 Ounces Chicken Broth, Low Sodium

Fennel Fronds for Garnish

Orange Slices for Garnish

Directions:

Thin your pork tenderloin by spreading them between parchment sheets and pounding with a mallet.

Heat a skillet, and add in your oil. Place it over medium heat, and cook your fennel seeds for three minutes.

Add the pork to the pan, cooking for an additional three minutes per side.

Transfer your pork to a platter before setting it to the side, and add in your fennel and onion.

Cook for five minutes, and then place the vegetables to the side.

Pour in your broth and wine, and bring it to a boil over high heat. Cook until the liquid has reduced by half.

Return your pork to the skillet, and cook for another five minutes.

Stir in your onion mixture, covering again. Cook for two more minutes, and serve warm.

Nutrition:

Calories: 276 Protein: 23.4 Grams Fat: 24 Grams Carbs: 14 GramsSodium: 647 mg Cholesterol: 49 mg

42.   Beefy Fennel Stew

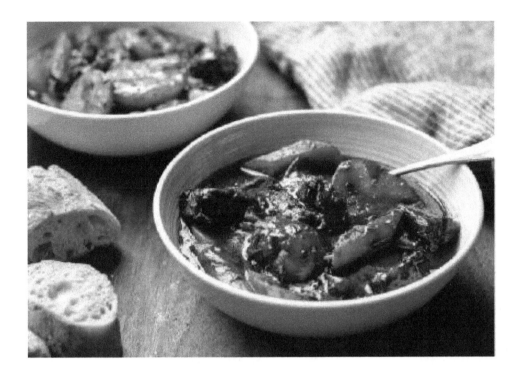

Preparation Time: 1 Hour 40 Minutes

Cooking Time: 1 Hour 40 Minutes

Servings: 4

Ingredients: 1 lb. Lean Beef, Boneless & Cubed - 2 Tablespoons Olive Oil - ½ Fennel Bulb, Sliced

3 Tablespoons All Purpose Flour - 3 Shallots, Large & Chopped - ¾ Teaspoon Black Pepper, Divided

2 Thyme Sprigs, Fresh - 1 Bay Leaf - ½ Cup Red Wine - 3 Cups Vegetable Stock

4 Carrots, Peeled & Sliced into 1 Inch Pieces - 4 White Potatoes, Large & Cubed

18 Small Boiling Onions, Halved - 1/3 Cup Flat Leaf Parsley, Fresh & Chopped

3 Portobello Mushrooms, Chopped

Directions:

Get out a shallow container and add in your flour. Dredge the beef cubes through it, shaking off the excess flour. Get out a saucepan and add in your oil, heating it over medium heat.

Add your beef, and cook for five minutes. Add in your fennel and shallots, cooking for seven minutes. Stir in your pepper, bay leaf and thyme. Cook for a minute more. Add your beef to the pan with your stock and wine. Boil it and reduce it to a simmer. Cover, cooking for forty-five minutes.

Add in your onions, potatoes, carrots and mushrooms. Cook for another half hour, which should leave your vegetables tender. Remove the thyme sprigs and bay leaf before serving warm. Garnish with parsley.

Nutrition: Calories: 244 Protein: 21 Grams Fat: 8 Grams Carbs: 22.1 Grams Sodium: 587 mg

Cholesterol: 125 mg

43.   Currant Pork Chops

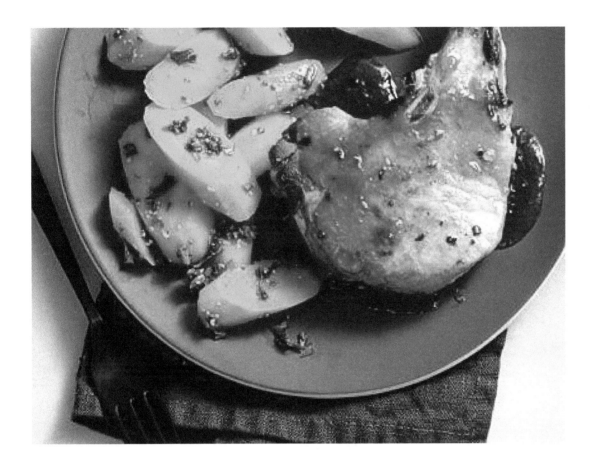

Preparation Time: 30 Minutes

Cooking Time: 30 Minutes

Servings: 6

Ingredients: 2 Tablespoons Dijon Mustard - 6 Pork Loin Chops, Center Cut -
2 Teaspoons Olive Oil

1/3 Cup Wine Vinegar - ¼ Cup Black Currant Jam - 6 Orange Slices - 1/8
Teaspoon Black Pepper

Directions:

Start by mixing your mustard and jam together in a bowl.

Get out a nonstick skillet, and grease it with olive oil before placing it over
medium heat. Cook your chops for five minutes per side, and then top with a
tablespoon of the jam mixture. Cover, and allow it to cook for two minutes.
Transfer them to a serving plate.

Pour your wine vinegar in the same skillet, and scape the bits up to deglaze the pan, mixing well. Drizzle this over your pork chops. Garnish with pepper and orange slices before serving warm.

Nutrition:

Calories: 265

Protein: 25 Grams

Fat: 6 Grams

Carbs: 11 Grams

Sodium: 120 mg Cholesterol: 22 mg

44.   Spicy Tomato Shrimp

Preparation Time: 35 Minutes

Cooking Time: 35 Minutes

Servings: 6

Ingredients:

¾ lb. Shrimp, Uncooked, Peeled & Deveined

2 Tablespoons Tomato Paste

½ Teaspoon Garlic, Minced

½ Teaspoon Olive Oil

1 ½ Teaspoons Water

½ Teaspoon Oregano, Chopped

½ Teaspoon Chipotle Chili Powder

Directions:

Rinse and dry the shrimp before setting them to the side.

Get out a bowl and mix your tomato paste, water, chili powder, oil, oregano and garlic. Spread this over your shrimp, and make sure they're coated on both sides.

Marinate for about twenty minutes or until you're ready to grill. Preheat a gas grill to medium heat, and then grease the grate with oil. Place it six inches from the heat source. Skewer the shrimp, and for four minutes per side. Serve warm.

Nutrition:

Calories: 185

Protein: 16.9 Grams

Fat: 1 Gram

Carbs: 12.4 Grams

Sodium: 394 mg

Cholesterol: 15 mg

45.   Beef Stir Fry

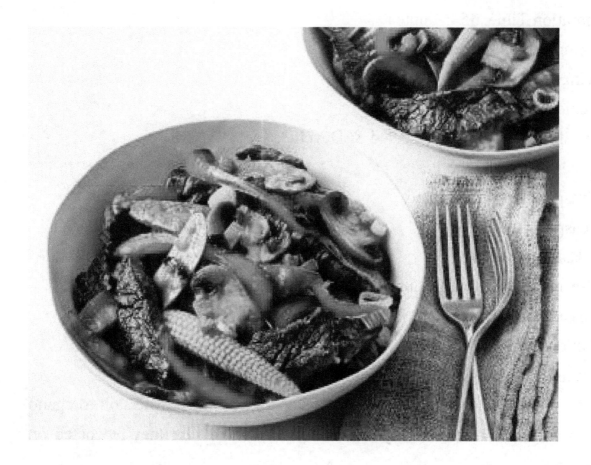

Preparation Time: 40 Minutes

Cooking Time: 40 Minutes

Servings: 4

Ingredients: 1 Head Broccoli Chopped into Florets - 1 Red Bell Pepper, Sliced Thin

1 ½ Cups Brown Rice - 2 Scallions, Sliced Thin - 2 Tablespoons Sesame Seeds

¼ Teaspoon Black Pepper

1 lb. Flank Steak, Sliced Thin

2 Tablespoons Canola Oil

¾ Cup Stir Fry Sauce

Directions:

Start by heating your oil in a large wok over medium-high heat. Add in your steak, seasoning with pepper. Cook for four minutes or until crisp. Remove it from the skillet.

Place your broccoli in the skillet and cook for four minutes. Toss occasionally. It should be tender but crisp.

Put your steak back in the skillet, and pour in your sauce. Allow it to simmer for three minutes.

Serve over rice with sesame seeds and scallions.

Nutrition:

Calories: 408 Protein: 31 Grams Fat: 18 Grams

Carbs: 36 Grams Sodium: 461 mg Cholesterol: 57 mg

Chapter 14   Dessert Recipes

46.   Rice Pudding with Mango

Preparation time: 55 minutes

Cooking time: 55 minutes

Servings: 4

Ingredients:

1 teaspoon vanilla extract

1/2 teaspoon ground cinnamon

2 tablespoons sugar

1 cup vanilla soy milk

Peeled and chopped mango (optional)

1 medium ripe mango (peeled, sliced, and mashed)

1 cup long-grain brown rice (uncooked)

1/4 teaspoon salt

2 cups water

Directions:

Put water and salt in a pan over medium-high flame. Bring to a boil. Add rice. Turn heat to low and cover the pan. Simmer for 40 minutes. Add mashed mango, cinnamon, sugar, and milk. Continue cooking for 15 minutes while occasionally stirring.

Turn off the heat and add vanilla.

You can have this hot or cold. Top with chopped mango, if preferred, before serving.

Nutrition:

Calories: 275

Protein: 4.66 g

Fat: 2.58 g

Carbohydrates: 43.34 g
Sodium: 176 mg

47.   Light Choco Pudding

Preparation time: 32 minutes

Cooking time: 32 minutes

Servings: 4

Ingredients:

1 teaspoon vanilla extract

2 cups chocolate soy milk

1/8 teaspoon salt

2 tablespoons baking cocoa

2 tablespoons sugar

3 tablespoons cornstarch

Directions:

Put milk in a pan over medium flame. Add salt, cocoa, sugar, and cornstarch. Mix until thick and bubbly. Turn heat to low and continue cooking for 2 minutes.

Turn off the heat, add vanilla and allow to cool while stirring every now and then. Transfer to a bowl, cover and refrigerate for 30 minutes before serving.

Nutrition:

Calories: 127

Protein: 4.38 g

Fat: 1.49 g

Carbohydrates: 27.14 g

Sodium: 112 mg

48.   Peach Tart

Preparation time: 52 minutes

Cooking time: 52 minutes

Servings: 8

Ingredients: 1 cup all-purpose flour

1/4 teaspoon ground nutmeg

3 tablespoons sugar

1/4 cup butter (softened)

For the filling:

1/4 cup sliced almonds

1/8 teaspoon almond extract

1/4 teaspoon ground cinnamon

Whipped cream (optional)

2 tablespoons all-purpose flour

1/3 cup sugar

2 pounds peaches (peeled and sliced)

Directions:

Put butter, sugar, and butter in a bowl. Mix until fluffy. Add flour and beat until combined. Transfer to a tart pan and firmly spread and press to the bottom. Put on a baking sheet in the oven's middle rack. Bake in a preheated oven at 375 degrees F for 12 minutes. Leave to cool.

Put peaches in a bowl. Add almond extract, cinnamon, flour, and sugar. Toss to coat. Scoop on top of the crust. Add chopped almonds on top. Put on the lower rack of the oven and bake for 40 minutes. Allow to cool.

Serve as is or you can also opt to top it with whipped cream.

Nutrition:

Calories: 222

Protein: 2.61 g

Fat: 6.14 g
Carbohydrates: 47.84 g
Sodium: 46 mg

49.   Yogurt Parfait with Lime and Grapefruit

Preparation time:

Cooking time:

Servings: 6

Ingredients:

3 tablespoons honey

2 tablespoons lime juice

2 teaspoons grated lime zest

Fresh mint leaves (torn)

4 cups plain yogurt (reduced-fat)

4 large red grapefruit

Directions:

Cut a small part of each grapefruit's top and bottom. Make them stand on a cutting board. Cut off peel and gently slice through the membrane of the fruit's segment to get the fruit.

Put juice, lime zest, and yogurt in a bowl. Arrange half of the grapefruit in 6 parfait glasses. Top each glass with half of the yogurt mixture. Repeat until you have no more fruit and yogurt mixture left. Top each glass with honey and mint.

Nutrition:

Calories: 207

Protein: 7.12 g

Fat: 5.53 g

Carbohydrates: 34.71 g

Sodium: 115 mg

50. Fruit and Nut Bites

Preparation time: 1 hour

Cooking time: 0 minute

Servings: 4 dozen

Ingredients:

1 cup pistachios (toasted and finely chopped)

1 cup dried cherries (finely chopped)

2 cups dried apricots (finely chopped)

1/4 cup honey

1/4 teaspoon almond extract

3 3/4 cups sliced almonds (divided)

Directions:

Put 1 1/4 cups of almonds in a food processor. Pulse until chopped. Transfer to a bowl and set aside.

Process 2 1/2 cups almonds in a food processor until chopped. Gradually add extract and honey as you process. Transfer to a bowl. Add cherries and apricots. Divide into 6 and shape them into thick rolls. Wrap in plastic and leave in the fridge for an hour.

Remove plastic and cut each roll to 1 1/2 inch piece. Roll half of them in pistachios. Roll the other half in almonds. Wrap each piece in waxed paper and store in an airtight container.

Nutrition:

Calories: 86

Protein: 9.22 g

Fat: 14.95 g

Carbohydrates: 72.36 g

Sodium: 15 mg

Chapter 15   28 Day Meal Plan

Days	Breakfast	Lunch/Dinner	Snacks
1	Sunny-Side up Baked Eggs with Swiss chard, Feta, and Basil	Cheesy Black Bean Wraps	Fennel Sauce Tenderloin
2	Harissa Shakshuka with Bell Peppers and Tomatoes	Arugula Risotto	Beefy Fennel Stew
3	Egg in a "Pepper Hole" with Avocado	Vegetarian Stuffed Eggplant	Currant Pork Chops
4	Polenta with Sautéed Chard and Fried Eggs	Vegetable Tacos	Spicy Tomato Shrimp
5	Smoked Salmon Egg Scramble with Dill and Chives	Tuscan Stew	Beef Stir Fry
6	Eggs Benedict	Simple Pasta Limon	Rice Pudding with Mango
7	Fruit Smoothie	Baked Salmon with Dill 'n Garlic	Light Choco Pudding
8	Green Smoothie	Pan-Fried Kale Falafel	Peach Tart
9	Homemade Bacon	Stir-Fried Brussels Sprouts Korean Style	Yogurt Parfait with Lime and Grapefruit

10	Oatmeal Pancakes	Tuna-Pasta Salad	Fruit and Nut Bites
11	Sunny-Side up Baked Eggs with Swiss chard, Feta, and Basil	Red Lentil and Cauliflower Curry	Homemade Spinach Artichoke Dip
12	Harissa Shakshuka with Bell Peppers and Tomatoes	Black Bean Soup	Pumpkin Walnut Cookie
13	Egg in a "Pepper Hole" with Avocado	Avocado-Orange Grilled Chicken	Choco-Chip Cookies with Walnuts and Oatmeal
14	Polenta with Sautéed Chard and Fried Eggs	American Cheese Over Herbed Portobello Mushrooms	Potato Casserole
15	Smoked Salmon Egg Scramble with Dill and Chives	Garden Salad with Oranges 'n Olives	Cornbread with Southern Twist
16	Eggs Benedict	Roasted Vegetables with Polenta	Deviled Eggs Guac Style
17	Fruit Smoothie	Herbed and Spiced Grilled Eggplant	Buffalo Chicken Dip
18	Green Smoothie	Low Sodium Shepherd's Pie	Ricotta and Pomegranate Bruschetta
19	Homemade Bacon	Dijon Mustard and Lime Marinated Shrimp	Crab Stuffed Mushrooms

20	Oatmeal Pancakes	Cheesy Black Bean Wraps	Sour Cream and Onion Dip Carrot Sticks
21	Sunny-Side up Baked Eggs with Swiss chard, Feta, and Basil	Arugula Risotto	Fennel Sauce Tenderloin
22	Harissa Shakshuka with Bell Peppers and Tomatoes	Vegetarian Stuffed Eggplant	Beefy Fennel Stew
23	Egg in a "Pepper Hole" with Avocado	Vegetable Tacos	Currant Pork Chops
24	Polenta with Sautéed Chard and Fried Eggs	Tuscan Stew	Spicy Tomato Shrimp
25	Smoked Salmon Egg Scramble with Dill and Chives	Simple Pasta Limon	Beef Stir Fry
26	Eggs Benedict	Baked Salmon with Dill 'n Garlic	Rice Pudding with Mango
27	Fruit Smoothie	Pan-Fried Kale Falafel	Light Choco Pudding
28	Green Smoothie	Stir-Fried Brussels Sprouts Korean Style	Peach Tart

Conclusion

If you are reading this book, then you have already taken an important step by making your health, or the health of a loved one, a priority—congratulations! One of the biggest parts of becoming healthy is taking control and becoming informed. This book will make it easy for you to embrace a diet proven to lower blood pressure, cholesterol, and the risk for a number of chronic diseases. And you can start all this right now. Change your thinking about dieting, evolve from limiting yourself to thinking about what you can add to your diet, and what you can add to your life. Find your inner motivation, whether it is to be able to keep up with your grandchildren or to finally walk that half-marathon—harness your inner drive and make the commitment to optimize your health. If you stick with it and believe in yourself, you're going to reach your goal. Get ready to embrace the new you. I believe in you.

Remember the DASH is designed not for losing weight, but to lower blood pressure. It does this by balancing your mineral intake. Sodium promotes fluid retention and raises blood pressure, but other minerals like potassium and magnesium have the opposite effect. You do need salt of course, but since most Americans consume far too much sodium, the balance between all these important minerals is disrupted, leading to high blood pressure. The DASH diet addresses this issue.

The DASH diet also includes a simplified system based on numbers of portions per day, rather than counting calories which makes it easy to follow.

So by combining the two diets, we get the best approach possible to improved health and weight loss. We get the DASH approach to lowering blood pressure with its simple easy-to-follow portion approach, together with the heart-healthy fats of the Mediterranean diet.